Praise for
Finally Full, Finally Slim

"In FINALLY FULL, FINALLY SLIM, Lisa Young gives portion control the respect it deserves, while respecting the challenges of getting portions right without going hungry. Providing a comprehensive array of empowering strategies to make your diet better and turn the 'right' amount of food into 'enough,' this book is a feast of information—perfectly spiced with both humor and wisdom."

—David L. Katz, MD, MPH, founder of True Health Initiative, author of *The Truth about Food*

"FINALLY FULL, FINALLY SLIM tackles one of the biggest challenges to reaching and keeping a healthy weight—portion sizes. The supersizing of restaurant meals, sodas, burgers, fries, cookies, shakes, candy, and more has caused a national epidemic of portion distortion. Young's book teaches people how to normal-size their meals…and, eventually, their bodies."

—Margo G. Wootan, DSc, vice president for nutrition, Center for Science in the Public Interest

"Dr. Young broke new ground with readers with her first book, *The Portion Teller*. Understanding how portion sizes can easily be underestimated and derail your diet is critical to healthy eating and weight control. In her new book, Dr. Young teaches readers how portion control, mindful eating, and other life patterns can positively and permanently impact eating behaviors. Recommendations based on time-tested research help readers to actively make adjustments to their eating habits for a healthier lifestyle."

—Charles Platkin, PhD, JD, MPH, editor of DietDetective.com and executive director of the Hunter College NYC Food Policy Center

"Living a slim life is not about diet. It's about smart, educated enjoyment of food and the healthy lifestyle that goes with it. Lisa's advice and strategies make it easy to start and stay on a path to living a slim life."

—Sarah Hiner, CEO, Bottom Line Inc., publishers of *Bottom Line/Personal, Bottom Line/Health,* BottomLineInc.com

"Dr. Lisa Young's new book, FINALLY FULL, FINALLY SLIM, tackles THE biggest issue in weight loss: portion control. Her science-based approach offers readers realistic ways to get control of their portion sizes, without feeling deprived. If you struggle to lose weight, this book is for you."

—Nicole Avena, PhD, author of *What to Eat When You're Pregnant*

"When it comes to controlling your portions to manage your weight, Lisa Young really knows her stuff! She'll show you how to limit your portions of certain foods while letting loose with others (like fruits and veggies), while maintaining a healthy diet. This way, you can enjoy the foods you like and get (or stay) slim—without feeling deprived. It's a smart and simple approach that works for life!"

—Stacey Colino, award-winning health writer

"FINALLY FULL, FINALLY SLIM is smart, accessible, and a good read—three essentials if you're looking to make a change in your life." —Joe Dziemianowicz, *NY Daily News*

Finally Full, Finally Slim

Also by Lisa R. Young, PhD, RDN

The Portion Teller:
Smartsize Your Way to Permanent Weight Loss

The Portion Teller Plan:
The No-Diet Reality Guide to Eating, Cheating,
and Losing Weight Permanently

Finally Full, Finally Slim

30 Days to
Permanent Weight Loss
One Portion at a Time

Lisa R. Young, PhD, RDN

CENTER
STREET

New York   Nashville

Copyright © 2019 by Lisa R. Young

Cover design by Edward A. Crawford. Cover photography by Getty Images. Cover copyright © 2019 by Hachette Book Group, Inc.

Center Street
Hachette Book Group
1290 Avenue of the Americas, New York, NY 10104
centerstreet.com
twitter.com/centerstreet

First Edition: January 2019

Center Street is a division of Hachette Book Group, Inc. The Center Street name and logo are trademarks of Hachette Book Group, Inc.

The publisher is not responsible for websites (or their content) that are not owned by the publisher.

The Hachette Speakers Bureau provides a wide range of authors for speaking events. To find out more, go to www.HachetteSpeakersBureau.com or call (866) 376-6591.

Gag quotes used in chapters "Gaining Weight? It's Your Portions!" and "Day #8" courtesy Glasbergen Cartoon Service.

Illustrations by Christopher Jiménez unless otherwise noted

Library of Congress Cataloging-in-Publication Data

Names: Young, Lisa R., author.
Title: Finally full, finally slim : 30 days to permanent weight loss one
    portion at a time / Lisa R. Young, PhD, RDN.
Other titles: Portion teller plan.
Description: First edition. | Nashville : Center Street, 2019. | Revision of:
    Portion teller plan / Lisa R. Young. c2005. 1st pbk. ed. | Includes
    bibliographical references and index.
Identifiers: LCCN 2018029927| ISBN 9781478993025 (hardcover) | ISBN
    9781549199868 (audio download) | ISBN 9781478993018 (ebook)
Subjects: LCSH: Weight loss. | Reducing diets. | Food portions. | Nutrition.
Classification: LCC RM222.2 .Y683 2019 | DDC 613.2/5—dc23
LC record available at https://lccn.loc.gov/2018029927

ISBNs: 978-1-4789-9302-5 (hardcover), 978-1-4789-9301-8 (ebook)

Printed in the United States of America

LSC-C

10 9 8 7 6 5 4 3 2

To Mom and Dad,

for teaching me to never give up

and that anything worth having in life

is worth fighting for

Contents

STAGE 3 **Your Habits**

STAGE 4 **Your Life**

Introduction

The second day of a diet is always easier than the first. By the second day, you're off it.

—Jackie Gleason

As a nutritionist, I am often asked, "What's the best way to lose weight?" People share with me the super restrictive (and often scary) plans they've tried or radical approaches they've heard about. When I mention *portion control*, they say, "Yes, you are right—portion sizes are too big, but it's difficult to eat less. It's easier to just omit an entire food group." Yet they still wonder how to lose weight and keep it off.

Many diet plans out there are only temporary fixes that leave us struggling with weight and obsessing about food. Portion control is different. You don't have to cut out any food groups. You just have to right-size your portions.

In *Finally Full, Finally Slim*, I teach you how to enjoy food as nature intended—by consuming healthy portions of foods from all of the food groups. I don't ask you to banish nutritious foods from your table or buy miracle ingredients. (There really are none!) You don't have to eat anything you don't like. You can eat three meals a day, with snacks in between. You'll possibly be eating more than you do now. You'll learn which foods you can pile on your plate (and still lose weight) and discover that any food can be eaten in the right portions. And you never have to be hungry. *Finally Full, Finally Slim* is about losing weight while feeling full—and not even realizing you're on a diet. It's about understanding the power behind portion control.

Food portions, if you haven't noticed, have gotten larger over the years. I first noticed this phenomenon in the 1980s. Muffins, bagels, and pasta dishes were ballooning in size, and a new word entered our vocabulary: supersize. When results of a national dietary intake survey reported that the average American gained 8 pounds in the 1980s (compared to 1 or 2 pounds per decade in the 1960s and 1970s), I was certain it was due to the size of our food portions. I felt compelled to explore my gut instinct and investigate just how big American food portions had become.

I became so passionate about expanding portion sizes in this country that for my doctoral dissertation at New York University, I traced the history of portion sizes and discovered just how widespread this trend had become—and the effect it was having on waistlines across the country. With the exception of sliced white bread, just about every food portion increased in size and without us even noticing—burgers, steaks, soft drinks, desserts, you name it. Worse, we started to believe that these large portions were normal. Americans were gaining weight at unprecedented rates. But no one in the nutrition field was talking—or writing—about portion sizes. Instead, everyone was debating fats versus carbohydrates.

In the early 2000s, I published a series of papers on the contribution of expanding portion sizes to the obesity epidemic. Since then, I've assumed the role of "portion advocate." I took my message mainstream in 2005 with *The Portion Teller Plan*, which exposed to the public what was happening to our portions and our health as a result. I also outlined the eating plan I used with many of my clients. The book struck a chord. I was featured in countless stories about the supersize phenomenon, which had crept up on us. By the reactions I was getting, it was clear that many people hadn't noticed the trend until they read my book. Today, portion control has become an entire field of study. It's that important when it comes to gaining and losing weight.

After *The Portion Teller Plan* came out, I received many requests for a follow-up how-to book. Readers, clients, and people who attended my lectures or saw me featured in the media were asking for a book to teach them *how* to deal with the supersize portions we are barraged with. Enter *Finally Full, Finally Slim*.

Finally Full, Finally Slim includes the latest research on portion sizes and puts this science into practice. In this book, I show you how to implement an eating plan that works for you. And because I believe that a solid weight-loss plan is about more than food, this book is also about lifestyle. Feeling vibrant and being able to button your jeans every day is dependent on the foods (and the amounts) you put in your body, but it's so much more. Weight loss and maintenance are equally dependent on your attitude. (Did you know that happy people make better food choices?) What you think and how you feel directly impact your bottom line, so to speak. Equally important are the state of your kitchen and the habits you've settled into—good and bad. *Finally Full, Finally Slim* not only helps you lose weight; it elevates how you connect with yourself and others. We'll look at the whole you: your mind-set, environment, habits, and life. All of these areas affect the number you see on the scale.

Finally Full, Finally Slim outlines a portion plan (the Plan), along with thirty days' worth of simple and exciting changes you can make. The first three chapters give you the skinny on portion sizes and the basics of the Plan itself. Once you've gotten through "The Finally Full, Finally Slim Portion Plan" chapter, you're ready to start losing weight. The remaining sections dig deeper by showing you how to approach life and still stay on the Plan. I give you some clever interventions, such as tricks to control portions and tips for how to avoid sneaky portion traps. You'll learn some simple strategies for how to better measure portions, dine out, snack, and even sleep, for instance, and see how making small changes in these areas can help you shed pounds. And, of course, you'll also get the scoop on *why* these changes work, inspiring you to keep moving forward.

You can read this book in several sittings or attack a section a day. It's up to you. But whatever you do, commit to the Plan for at least thirty days. This gives you a chance to see how well it works for you. Meanwhile, you can gradually incorporate the daily changes into your life. Picture it: a new, energetic you, feeling and looking better than ever. It's worth a month, wouldn't you agree?

My clients think so. I developed this program for my clients—adults and children, male and female—who had been struggling with extra pounds for years and believed they were incapable of losing weight. With a doctorate in nutrition and as a registered dietitian nutritionist, I've counseled and helped thousands of people lose weight and keep it off—simply by teaching them how to reportion their portions. And I can help you, too.

The desire to lose weight is nothing new. But our challenges now are greater than ever before. Food is readily available. All-day snacking has become the norm. And many people can financially afford to eat as much as they want. The result is that we've lost perspective regarding the purpose of food, which is to provide energy, to foster good health, and to be enjoyed.

I come from a family of what I like to call "volume eaters"—lovers of big portions. I can relate to people who love a full plate and who don't want to eat tiny portions. *Finally Full, Finally Slim* is not about staring at an empty plate—a dieter's worst fear. It's about seeing what you put on your plate from a fresh perspective.

After thirty years, I'm still researching portion sizes. With the number of obese Americans now at 40 percent, restaurants and food manufacturers are starting to wake up to the idea that oversized portions are contributing to our nation's—and now, the world's—obesity problems. More than ever, I'm convinced that awareness is the key to a healthy relationship with food. Once people realize how much portion sizes have grown over the past decades, and how they've been duped into believing more is better, they begin to see their meals in an entirely different light—and they begin to lose weight and keep it off.

When you learn how to resize your portions, you learn that you can enjoy food and still lose weight. You can eat out, enjoy special occasions, and indulge in a favorite treat. You can live life without obsessing about weight, and you don't have to restrict yourself or eat bizarre food combinations. Portion control outlives all fad diets because it isn't a diet. It's a lifestyle.

Gaining Weight?
It's Your Portions!

Don't slice the pizza! My diet says I'm only allowed to eat
one piece.

—Randy Glasbergen

Why are most people overweight—and becoming more so? Because
the world is working against us. Every day, we're surrounded by
food portions that we've been led to believe are normal. A small isn't
really a small anymore. Portion sizes are large, creating a sense of
what I like to call portion distortion, or perceiving oversized portions as standard or normal. And larger portions give us permission
to eat more.

Results of more than sixty high-quality studies found that people consistently consume more food when offered larger portions
compared to smaller portions.[1] When we go out to eat and the wait-
person delivers garlic bread and onion rings for starters, followed by
a meal consisting of a 12-ounce rib eye, an oversized baked potato,
and sautéed green beans, along with free refills on soda, we believe
that if the restaurant considers this a meal, it must be so. Recalling
our parents' orders to clean our plates, we dutifully finish up.

This phenomenon, known as "passive overeating," has been
linked to weight gain and obesity. In a recent and important study

by researchers at the University of Liverpool, participants who were served smaller portions chose to eat less at future meals when compared to participants who were given larger portions, prompting the researchers to confirm that the food industry could help to "normalize" our *perception* of how much food constitutes a reasonable portion by serving more appropriate portion sizes.[2]

Double or nothing: Exploding portion sizes

In the not-too-distant past, portion sizes were much smaller than they are today. Take a look at the infographic on page 3 from the Centers for Disease Control and Prevention, which is based on my research.

As I discussed in my previous book, *The Portion Teller Plan*, my research found that many food portions are *up to five times larger* than they were in the past. Sodas, burgers, French fries, bagels, muffins, and steaks are some examples of portions that have exploded in size. It's common to see 20-ounce steaks on restaurant menus and 64-ounce (that's ½ gallon!) sodas. A typical bagel or muffin has doubled in size and may now be the equivalent of five slices of bread.[3]

My more recent portion-size research compares a product's original size against 2002 and 2017 sizes. We're still seeing double and triple burgers, as well as beverages topping out at more than a quart. McDonald's has made some of the most progress, taking its supersize French fries and soda off the menu and slightly reducing the sizes of the other containers for these products. But the fast-food chain still offers several big products, including a quart-sized soda and a Double Quarter Pounder with Cheese, which weighs 10 ounces (and contains 750 calories!), and the Grand Mac, introduced in 2017, with more than 800 calories. The company also offers a series of Big Breakfast items, some weighing nearly 1 pound and containing more than 1,000 calories.

Decades ago, when a company first introduced a product to

THE NEW (AB)NORMAL

Portion sizes have been growing. So have we. The average restaurant meal today is more than four times larger than in the 1950s. And adults are, on average, 26 pounds heavier. If we want to eat healthy, there are things we can do for ourselves and our community: Order the smaller meals on the menu, split a meal with a friend, or, eat half and take the rest home. We can also ask the managers at our favorite restaurants to offer smaller meals.

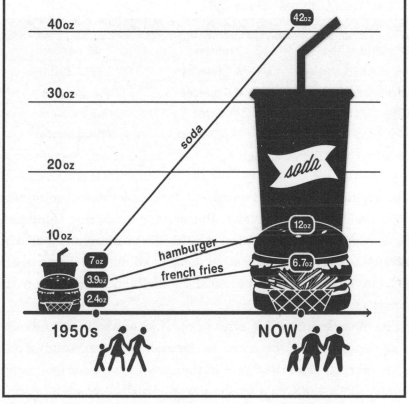

SOURCES: Young L, Nestle M. The contribution of expanding portions sizes to the US obesity epidemic. *Am J Public Health*. 2002;92(2):246–249; Young L, Nestle M. Portion sizes and obesity: responses of fast food companies. *J Public Health Policy*. 2007;28(2):238–248; CDC, Advance Data, No. 347, October 27, 2004; CDC, National Health Statistics Reports, No. 10, October 22, 2008.
Artwork: Centers for Disease Control and Prevention, 2012.

the market, it came in a one-size-fits-all package. Now we're seeing some products in as many as ten different sizes. Coca-Cola now offers six bottles ranging in size from 8 to 24 ounces, in addition to three different-sized cans, all marketed as single servings despite their size. The company has introduced a 7.5-ounce can of Coke, but it costs more than the 12-ounce can! Offering multiple sizes (most of them big) has been on the rise.

Portion Sizes: Original versus 2017

Product	Original Size	2017 Size
Budweiser, bottle	7 ounces	7–40 ounces
Burger King, sandwich	3.9 ounces	3.3–12.2 ounces
Hershey's bar	0.6 ounces	1.6–7 ounces
McDonald's soda	7 ounces	12–30 ounces
7-Eleven soda fountain	12–20 ounces	20–50 ounces

Information obtained from manufacturers and compiled by Lisa R. Young, PhD, RDN, 2017.

In a nation with a predominantly more-is-better mentality, bigger portions mean better sales. But at what cost? The Centers for Disease Control and Prevention recently dropped a bombshell when they announced that nearly 40 percent of adults and 19 percent of youths in the United States are obese—the highest rates the nation has ever seen.[4]

The increase in portion sizes goes hand in hand with increases in calorie intake and obesity rates. Americans are consuming more calories per day than they were in the past. In fact, our food supply provides about 4,000 calories per person per day—twice as much as most of us need and a considerable increase from the 3,200 calories per person per day back in 1980. Some of the calories in the food supply are lost to food waste and spoilage, but nevertheless, the data is useful for assessing trends in how much we eat.[5]

Research conducted by Tufts University found that casual

sit-down and fast-food chain restaurant meals are supersized, whether they say so or not. The average meal contained 1,200 calories, which is more than half of what you should eat in an entire day. American, Italian, and Chinese meals tended to have the most calories, averaging 1,500 each.[6] Think your local café is a healthier choice? Probably not. Nine out of ten nonchain restaurants also exceeded the calorie recommendations for a single meal. Every year, the Center for Science in the Public Interest, a consumer advocacy group in Washington, DC, grants Xtreme Eating Awards to "honor" oversized dishes chock-full of calories. Among their most recent awards were menu items that topped 2,500 calories.[7]

Outlandish portion sizes mean that we're eating far more calories than we realize—and most certainly more than we need. Here's a look at what some restaurants and cafés consider a normal portion size:

- Mocha coffee, 330 calories
- Bagel, 400 calories
- Chocolate chip cookie, 400 calories
- Big Mac, 540 calories
- Beef and broccoli, 700 calories
- Personal pan pizza (to serve one), 720 calories
- Rib eye steak (12 ounces—many cuts are larger than this!), 800 calories
- Cheese quesadilla, 830 calories
- Greek salad, 900 calories
- Double Whopper sandwich with cheese, 930 calories
- Lasagna, 950 calories
- Spaghetti with meatballs, 1,200 calories
- Popcorn (large) with butter at a movie theater, 1,200 calories
- Chorizo fiesta omelet, 1,300 calories
- General Tso's chicken, 1,750 calories
- Breakfast burrito, 2,700 calories

It's not only eating out where we are easily fooled. Food packaging throws us for a loop as well. If you take the time to read the label on a potato chip package, you may be relieved to find they're only 160 calories a serving. But you probably don't realize that a serving is just fifteen chips or so. Mimicking the huge bowls pictured on cereal packaging, many people pour 2–3 cups of cereal into a bowl, versus the 1 cup most nutritionists recommend.

You're underestimating how many calories you're eating

With many of us growing up with oversized portions as the norm, we have lost all sense of how many calories we're eating. Oversized portions contain far more calories than you might realize. A small hamburger may contain 300 calories, while a larger one (what we think of as an acceptable portion) can easily contain 1,000 or more. A medium soda at the movie theater is the equivalent of 3 or 4 servings, containing 300 or 400 (or more!) calories.[8]

While it seems obvious that large portions have more calories than small portions, many people—even health-conscious people—routinely underestimate the difference. When I asked the nearly one hundred college students in my introductory nutrition class at New York University how many calories were in an 8-ounce soda compared to a 64-ounce soda, 70 percent underestimated the proportional increase in calories. An 8-ounce serving of soda contains 100 calories, so a 64-ounce serving contains 800 calories. Most students, however, guessed the number of calories to be closer to 300, not 800!

Is the health-food craze contributing to weight gain?

Today's emphasis on whole foods may be good news for overall nutrient intake, but you might just give yourself permission to overeat foods just because they're healthy. My client Amy, for instance, is a devotee of the Paleo diet, which focuses on eating whole, unprocessed foods and omitting dairy and grains. She came to me baffled that she could not lose weight. She had cut out processed foods and

SUBTLE INFLUENCES

Here are just a few of the studies that reveal that the size of the portion offered, the size of its container, the number of portions offered, and other factors all affect how much we eat and how well we estimate our calorie consumption.

- People ate more pizza when the pie was cut into 8 slices compared to 16 slices. (We eat in units, and when served a unit of food—say, a slice of pizza, a cookie, or a sandwich—we tend to eat the entire thing, regardless of its size.)[9]

- When served a large sandwich, people ate about one-third to one-half more than when given a smaller one.[10]

- In a real-life work setting, people exposed to a larger lunch for six months ate significantly more calories and gained weight when compared to those who received a smaller lunch.[11]

- Bottle-fed babies gained more weight when their parents used larger bottles to feed them![12]

- Nearly 25 percent of people underestimated the calorie content of a meal by at least 500 calories when presented with a larger portion![13]

- While more than 75 percent of people realized they ate more after receiving a large portion, they underestimated how much they ate by 25 percent.[14]

- People underestimated the calories in foods they perceived as healthy or low fat and ate up to 50 percent more after seeing a label with a low-fat claim.[15]

snacked on nuts and avocados. She had no idea how much she was eating—just that she was eating the healthy foods permitted on the diet. When Amy tracked her food intake and told me she consumed two avocados and about 1 cup of nuts a day in snacks alone, mystery solved. Nuts and avocados are healthy foods—but eat too much of them and you'll gain weight.

Eating too much of a good thing is still eating too much. We often take this one step further and eat too much of foods we *perceive* as healthy. Our perceptions usually stem from clever marketing claims. There's even a term used to describe these claims: health halos. We automatically think that marketing labels such as "all natural" or "low fat" mean a product is good for us, even though it may have more calories or sugar than similar products. Health halos such as "organic," "gluten-free," and "sugar-free" distract us to the point where we ignore portion sizes and sometimes nutrition quality. Low-fat cookies are still cookies and gluten-free crackers are still crackers. Eat too much of them and you'll gain weight.

Fighting back by resetting the norm

The US Food and Drug Administration (FDA), for the first time since 1993, recently revamped the Nutrition Facts food label and updated the serving sizes listed on packaged foods and beverages. Many of the serving sizes have increased, for instance, to better reflect the amount most Americans actually eat. This is important because consumers often do not pay attention to the serving size when reading food labels and may, therefore, believe they are eating fewer calories than they really are.[16]

Updating food-label serving sizes is a step in the right direction. But we also need to reset the norm. Doing away with big portions is ultimately the best answer. We've made some progress since my research first came out in 2002, but more advocacy still needs to be done.

In *Finally Full, Finally Slim*, you'll learn how to fight back against this more-is-better environment. I teach you how to reportion your portions so you can lose weight, and keep it off, while eating the foods you love. No suffering and no starving required. I promise that you will never have to stare at an empty plate. Just the opposite. You'll eat healthy portions of all foods and unlimited portions of some so that you stay full while you lose weight. Eating thoughtful portions becomes surprisingly automatic once you get used to it. You won't have to think about what or how much to eat—your new habits will become part of you and require no effort to maintain. So let's get started!

Supersize This, Downsize That

"Enough" is a feast.
—Buddhist proverb

If you're anything like my clients, you want to know what you're getting yourself into: What are your new go-to foods? What will you have to give up? How much effort will it be? How much can you eat? I'm not going to sugarcoat it. I do have some rules, or really guidelines. But they are about as flexible as an overcooked noodle. So allow me to give you the scoop on some of the details of the Plan by answering some of the most common questions I hear from my clients.

Q: When I hear "portion control," I think "tiny." Will I be staring at an empty plate?
A: Just the opposite.

My definition of portion control is about eating big portions of foods with small calorie counts (fruits and vegetables) and normal (not oversized) portions of other healthy foods, while shifting away from unhealthy choices. The portions I recommend of certain foods may be smaller or larger than your current portions, so you'll be making some adjustments. I also give you a wild card: You are free to eat as many fruits and vegetables (freebies) as you want, whenever you want. Freebies are relatively low in calories, and they contain a lot of fiber, which helps you feel full. Being able to eat as many as you want means you never have to stare at an empty plate. (We'll cover freebies in depth in Day #13: Fill Up on Freebies, page 130.)

If I had to sum it up in a sentence: The Plan is about knowing

BUT I HATE VEGETABLES!

Every now and then, I get a client who claims she hates vegetables— everything from the texture to the taste. When someone tells me she rejects all vegetables, I have to believe she has prematurely closed the door on one of life's greatest pleasures. I'm not sure how this happens. Maybe when she hears "vegetables," all she can think of is the soggy, limp boiled broccoli from her high school cafeteria days. But replacing those unwanted memories with some new experiences usually does the trick. So I suggest she get creative.

If you don't like steamed (or boiled) broccoli, put broccoli slaw in a salad. Sauté it with a little olive oil, garlic, and lemon or add it to a soup. Not a fan of cauliflower's texture? Experiment with cauliflower rice, which is light and fluffy. Think zucchini's only good for composting? Spiral it to make zoodles, or veggie pasta. Cook it lightly with fresh tomato sauce and Parmesan cheese and you'll think you're eating traditional spaghetti. For a totally different taste, make a smoothie by blending fruits and veggies.

The Internet puts a gazillion healthy recipes at your fingertips. Explore. Have fun. Try a small bit of a veggie you haven't eaten in years. If you don't like the texture, change it. (Changing texture can also change taste.) If you don't like the taste, liven it up. You don't have to fall in love with every vegetable. My vegetable-rejecting clients almost always come around to liking at least a few vegetables, prepared just their way, and that's good enough.

which foods you can supersize and which to downsize. When it comes to food choices on the Plan, a common theme is low-calorie, nutrient-rich foods teeming with vitamins, minerals, and fiber. Most of my clients are surprised to see how much they can eat on the Plan. Many even tell me they don't know how they could possibly squeeze in so much food in a day. They think they're eating more food, but really it's just healthier, more satisfying food than they're used to eating. And, much to their surprise, they are eating fewer calories.

Q: Do I have to change what I eat?
A: It depends on how healthy your diet is now.

If you enjoy foods from the Mediterranean diet (which is heavy in whole foods such as fruits and veggies, fish, legumes, and whole grains and light on meats and heavily processed foods), for example, more power to you. You'll probably just need to size up your portions. Love fruit, chickpeas, and corn on the cob? I've got you covered. Vegan, gluten-free? Fine by me, as long as you're cognizant of nutrition, balance, and health halos, which you'll read about later (see Day #4: Debunk Health Halos, page 75). Unless your diet regularly consists of sodas, fast-food hamburgers, fries, and double hot fudge sundaes, or is otherwise nutritionally unsound, I'm not necessarily going to ask you to change what you eat. Only how much. And sometimes, how often.

I will suggest that you swap out white for whole-grain bread because it's a healthier choice. I like to think of it as shifting from less healthy to more healthy. You'll hardly notice these small changes, yet they make a big difference over time. I won't ever, though, ask you to give up starchy vegetables such as potatoes and sweet potatoes but suggest that you prepare them so they offer the maximum benefit with the lowest calorie count—maybe roasted or baked in their jackets instead of deep-fried, for instance. The more you get into the

Plan, the more you'll start thinking in terms of "this is better than that," and you'll quickly fall in love with these types of changes. Not only will you see the results, but you'll feel them as well.

Q: Do I have to control my portions forever?

A: Portion control is a lifestyle, not a diet.

Once you get used to eating healthy portions, they will feel normal. You'll wonder how you ate large portions before. As long as you make smart, healthy food choices most (about 80 percent) of the time, you can splurge some (about 20 percent) of the time. I believe strongly in this 80/20 rule, which is common in lifestyle plans. It's unrealistic to think that you can never eat your favorite treat or that you have to crunch only on carrot sticks at a party. My only request is that you do your best to plan your cheats and write them down in your Portion Tracker so they don't become 50 percent of your choices. We'll cover everything you need to know about the Portion Tracker in Day #2: Write It before You Bite It (see page 56).

Q: What about coffee?

A: Yes! You can keep your morning cup of joe.

Consider black coffee or coffee with low-fat or fat-free milk or milk swaps such as unsweetened almond milk to be the best option. Even cappuccino with low-fat milk is fine, but hold the cream. If you put sugar in your coffee, try substituting cinnamon, vanilla, nutmeg, and even turmeric. Or, if you need to dress your coffee up every day, ask yourself whether you even like it to begin with. An alternative is to drink herbal teas—or green tea if you need a caffeine boost.

Q: On the days I exercise, can I increase my portions?

A: No, I recommend that you get creative with your snacks.

Snacks work wonders in getting you from a morning workout to lunch or through your evening workout and all the way to dinner. They curb hunger and boost energy, which is important whether you're doing yoga or going for a jog. Because I also encourage you to exercise regularly on this program, I want you to enjoy your workouts—not be too full or too hungry to participate. On the Plan, you can divvy up your servings any way you like, so use your servings to create healthy pre- and post-workout energy boosters.

Keep in mind that exercise doesn't burn as many calories as you might think. Its bigger benefit is that it turns on your body's healthy mode. After a good workout, you feel more in tune with your body, and cravings for junk food diminish. Exercise also helps reduce stress and improve mood. Stress eaters may find that exercise replaces stress eating. You'll find more about snacks and workouts in Day #24: Step It Up (see page 209).

Q: Do I need to give up carbs to lose weight?
A: No. You can eat carbs and lose weight on the Plan.

Carbohydrates are one of the most misunderstood pieces of the nutritional puzzle, and that's one reason I've devoted an entire day to them (see Day #6: Get Over Your Fear of Carbs, page 86). Here, I'll briefly explain that if you eat any fruits or vegetables, you have not given up carbs. Carbs are not just in breads and muffins and pizza crusts. They exist in many foods, including fruits, veggies, whole grains, milk, legumes, and nuts.

I've seen people order a large pizza pie, eat all of the cheese, and disregard the crust to avoid carbs. Why not just eat one slice of pizza and enjoy it with a salad and call it a fun, satisfying meal? Here's where the mind-set portion of the Plan comes into play: Eating only the top of the pizza to avoid a food group does not reflect a healthy food mentality. It reeks of deprivation and even fear. If you want pizza that much, give yourself permission to enjoy a slice. Adding a large salad gives you a heavy dose of satisfying nutrients, which will eliminate cravings for more than one slice.

Q: Is this a fad diet?
A: Not even close.

I like to look at the Plan as a foundation you can build any balanced diet on. It's more of a lifestyle plan than a diet, and it's a plan you can use with diets based on your lifestyle. Fad diets are sometimes excuses to avoid watching portion sizes. By cutting out entire food groups (such as grains and starchy vegetables) or filling up on miracle foods or ingredients (think: blending grass-fed butter into your coffee), many dieters believe they have permission to eat as much as they want, as long as they abide by the diet's guidelines. It's unlikely that they can live this way forever, though.

It is human nature to look for quick, magic fixes. Your high school reunion is two weeks away. You haven't lost 1 of the 10 pounds you swore you'd drop, so you give up starches at every meal for ten days. You lose some weight, impress the heck out of your old classmates, and then return to the same old eating habits that tipped the scale in the first place. If you continue to deny yourself grains and starchy vegetables at every meal, you might keep losing weight. But eventually you will feel the pangs of deprivation, and, well, your next reunion isn't for another ten years.

When weight loss is founded on unsustainable eating habits, weight loss is unsustainable. Diets that are too much work or leave you feeling deprived or stuck in a rut are not sustainable. On some level, turning to fad diets is a distraction. The answer to weight loss and health is right in front of you. It's been here all along: portion control. You, like all other dieters, have just been duped into believing that nothing could possibly be that basic. The core message of my Plan centers on portion size, and this message goes hand in hand with nutrition. Eat mindful portions of a wide variety of healthy foods and you'll lose weight and keep it off.

Q: How much effort do I have to put into this plan?
A: For thirty days, most of my clients put in slightly more effort than they would if they were not on a plan.

At the start, it's all about awareness. To get used to the portion sizes you should eat, the first thing you need to do is be aware of what and how much you are eating, as well as what healthy portions look like. Initially, you'll want to measure or eyeball what you put on your plate. You'll also want to record what you consume, in either an app, a small notebook, or the Portion Tracker supplied in this book (see page 285). All that transparency has a funny way of getting you to change your ways for the better.

There's no need to count calories or track grams of sugar and fat. I give you a wide variety of foods to choose from in the right portion sizes, so I have already done the math for you. Some of you may need to declutter your kitchen or get a sturdy pair of walking shoes. But that's about it. After thirty days, you'll be a proper portion professional. It'll be second nature, and you'll wonder why you didn't do it sooner.

DIETER'S DECREE

I will focus on what I can eat.

I will eat foods I enjoy.

I will focus on how I want to look and feel.

I will be open to enjoying foods from all the food groups.

I will swap out unhealthy foods for foods that are healthy and delicious.

I will leave troublesome (think: binge) foods at the grocery store.

I will burn calories daily by participating in sports or exercises I enjoy.

The right portion size is another way of saying *enough*—enough to fill your stomach and enough to keep your body fueled. Eating more than enough is adding unnecessary calories that can lead to weight gain. You could call it eating in moderation, but since your definition of moderation may be different from mine, the term really doesn't mean much unless it's defined. So I spell it out for you by showing you what realistic portion sizes look like.

Wherever you fall on the health-conscious scale (no pun intended), you will become one with the changes introduced to you throughout this book. Healthy choices will become automatic. You won't be consumed with this or that diet or second-guess your food choices. You'll be free to focus your thoughts and attention on areas of your life you didn't realize you were neglecting. A whole new world will open up to you. That's the power of portion control.

The Finally Full, Finally Slim Portion Plan

Food is an important part of a balanced diet.

—Fran Lebowitz

Here's where I unveil how much you can eat. As you already know, the Plan is about losing weight through food, not starvation, so your choices are plentiful. But first, just a few important notes.

Six food groups

You've got six food groups to work with:

Vegetables (nonstarchy)

Fruits

Starches (grains and starchy vegetables)

Fish, poultry, meat, and meat alternatives

Dairy

Fats

Bonus: treats and sweets (not a food group, per se, but I include it so you can feel good about satisfying a sweet tooth)

FINALLY FULL, FINALLY SLIM
PORTION PLATE

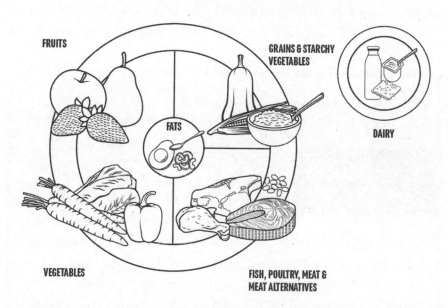

What's the difference between a serving and a portion?

Within each food group, you can have a certain number of servings. Think of a serving as a standard unit of measure: ½ cup, 3 ounces, or 1 tablespoon, for instance. Your portion is the amount of food you actually eat for a meal or snack. Portions may contain 1 or more servings. I spell out the standard serving sizes for foods in each food group (½ cup, for instance) along with the number of servings you can eat from the various food groups each day. The idea is that you can divvy up your servings as you like throughout the day, which gives you a great deal of flexibility.

Putting this into practice isn't nearly as complicated as it might sound. It quickly becomes second nature. For instance, you can enjoy

4–6 servings of starches (grains and starchy vegetables) every day. You might choose to have 1 cup of cooked oatmeal (2 servings) for breakfast, an open-faced sandwich with one slice of whole-grain toast (1 serving) for lunch, and half of a sweet potato (1 serving) with dinner on a given day. On another day, when you have plans to go out in the evening, you can save up all your starch servings for a hearty pasta dinner. You can mix and match any way you choose. It's entirely up to you.

Serving Sizes: Keep It Simple!

You may have heard of MyPlate, the US Department of Agriculture's (USDA's) nutrition education tool. MyPlate pictures a place setting with a plate and a glass of milk (or a serving of dairy) off to the side. The plate is sectioned into four food groups and shows Americans how much to eat from each food group for a healthy and balanced diet. My recommendations are similar to those in MyPlate but include several notable variations that are important for weight loss.

MyPlate, for instance, puts corn, potatoes, and other starchy vegetables in the vegetable food group, while I place them in starches, along with grains (except for French fries, which on the Plan are in the treats and sweets group). Corn and potatoes are among a dozen or so starchy vegetables, all of which have a calorie and carbohydrate content similar to grains. Likewise, MyPlate puts nuts in the protein group and avocados in the vegetable group, and I put them in fats because most of their calories come from fat. The USDA does not have a fats food group.[1]

How we refer to serving sizes also varies in some instances. USDA's MyPlate uses ounce or cup equivalents instead of serving sizes when referring to food amounts. For example, most people do not know what ounce equivalents for rice, pasta, and cereal look like, so I use the more customary cup measures. So keep it simple and follow the Plan. You'll be eating balanced, nutritious meals—and losing weight.

Serving ranges

Because we all come in different shapes and sizes with different weight-loss goals, I've provided some flexibility in the number of servings you can have from each food group. Where you fall in the range depends on several factors—namely, your age, gender, weight-loss goal, activity level, and appetite. To calculate your Finally Full, Finally Slim Number, or the ideal number of servings for you, consider all of the following.

Age. Metabolism, or the speed at which you burn calories, slows as you age. Several factors, including your body composition, age, and gender, determine your metabolism. As you age and lose lean body mass, your metabolism tends to slow down. If you're over fifty, start at the lower end of the range and see how you feel and how your weight loss progresses. Still growing? You're on the higher end.

Gender. Even with all other things being equal, men tend to have more lean body mass than women and, therefore, a faster metabolism. Men usually can eat more than women and still lose weight, so you guys can start at the top of the range.

Weight-loss goal. If your goal is to lose those stubborn 5 or 10 pounds, go for fewer servings. If you're on the heavier side, you can stick with a higher number of servings until you're at that 5- or 10-pound mark, at which point you can go low.

Activity level. If you exercise regularly and are on the go at work or at home with the kids, you've earned yourself a higher number of servings. If you are sedentary, your Finally Full, Finally Slim Number is on the lower side. As you increase your exercise, you might find you can increase your number of servings and still lose weight.

Appetite. Initially, avoid drastic changes in the amount of food you eat. If you are used to eating a lot more than the Plan recommends, give yourself the greatest number of servings allowed. If you are still hungry, eat more fruits and nonstarchy vegetables.

Determining your Finally Full, Finally Slim Number is not an exact science. As your exercise habits and weight-loss goals change, so might your Finally Full, Finally Slim Number. If you're not losing ½ or 1 pound per week, decrease your number of servings or increase your exercise. If you're feeling hungry or deprived, increase your servings—or, better yet, eat more fruits and veggies.

Now let's dive into the details for each food group in the Plan. We'll review how many servings of each food group you can have each day, what constitutes a serving, which foods you can always munch on, and which items you should turn down or "put a lid on." Foods listed in the "Go for it" section are great go-to foods. I encourage you to eat them. Just, as always, be mindful of your portions. Foods listed after "Put a lid on it" sections can be consumed; just tone it down by turning to them only on occasion and in small amounts. Even some foods in the freebie food groups (nonstarchy vegetables and fruits) have limits. So heed the advice to put a lid on these items. For more information, see Appendix A (page 245), which includes a comprehensive list of foods and serving sizes.

THE PLAN

VEGETABLES (NONSTARCHY)
FRUITS
STARCHES (GRAINS AND STARCHY VEGETABLES)
FISH, POULTRY, MEAT, AND MEAT ALTERNATIVES
DAIRY
FATS
TREATS AND SWEETS

VEGETABLES (NONSTARCHY)

How much?	Unlimited but at least 3 servings
What is a serving?	Vegetables, 1 cup
	Vegetable juice (low sodium), 1 cup (8 fluid ounces)
	Tomato sauce, ½ cup
Go for it:	A colorful assortment of fresh or frozen nonstarchy vegetables (for example, assorted greens, artichokes, broccoli, Brussels sprouts, carrots, cauliflower, cucumbers, eggplant, greens, kale, tomatoes, peppers, spaghetti squash, spinach, zucchini)
Put a lid on it:	Canned or frozen vegetables with added sauces or other ingredients

Remembering how many servings of nonstarchy veggies you can have is easy. On the Plan, you can eat as many as your heart desires. And your heart really does desire these foods, which are rich in vitamins and minerals and low in calories. Including plenty of veggies in your diet may protect you from a host of chronic diseases such as heart disease and diabetes. Filling up on them also safeguards you from overeating foods from other food groups. Veggies, among nature's most nutrient-dense foods, are jam-packed with fiber and water, which not only aid in digestion but leave you feeling full. And that's a good thing, since I intend on living up to my promise that you will never be hungry on this plan.

What the heck are nonstarchy vegetables?

The easiest way to answer this question is to tell you what starchy vegetables are, as there are far fewer of them: cassava, corn, green peas, parsnips, plantains, pumpkin, rutabagas, winter squash, potatoes, and sweet potatoes. These are perfectly fine veggies, and I encourage you to eat them. But if you want to lose weight, you can't eat unlimited quantities of them. They look like vegetables (because, well, they are vegetables), but their calorie—and carbohydrate—count is similar to that of bread and rice. For that reason, I group them with starches. We'll talk about them more in the starches section on page 28.

Otherwise, all nonstarchy vegetables are at your disposal anytime, any day. Everything from artichokes to zucchini. When choosing vegetables, let color be your guide. Different vitamins and antioxidants exist in the different color spectrums, so the more color and variety on your plate, the better. Look for dark greens (armed with nutrients that protect everything from your bones to your vision), bright reds (which contain the antioxidant lycopene), and oranges (which contain the antioxidant beta-carotene), all known powerhouses in the fight against chronic diseases. (The same holds true for fruit!) But I most definitely encourage you to eat all the colors of the rainbow and more—even white.

And take advantage of the many fun ways to bring more vegetables into your life: Bulk up pasta, rice, or a frozen dinner with carrots, mushrooms, or zoodles (spiraled zucchini); substitute cauliflower rice for rice; get in the habit of choosing salad as a side dish; and keep a supply of frozen vegetables in the freezer so you always have some on hand. Feel free to prepare your favorite veggies any way you like, but bear in mind that fat is not a food group you can consume in unlimited quantities (you'll read about how much fat you can have on pages 37–41). Whenever possible, eat your vegetables raw, steamed, roasted, microwaved, or sautéed with a drizzle of oil.

FRUITS

How much?	Whole fruit is unlimited, but at least 2 servings; for dried fruit, juice, and smoothies, see "Put a lid on it"
What is a serving?	Berries or melon, 1 cup
	Medium whole fruits (apple, orange, pear), 1
	Small whole fruits (kiwifruit, plum, fig), 2

Go for it:	A colorful assortment of fresh or frozen fruits
Put a lid on it:	Canned fruit in syrup, ½ cup
	Dried fruit, ¼ cup
	Fruit juice, 4 fluid ounces
	Fruit smoothies, 10–12 fluid ounces, limit to one a day (use no more than 1 cup fruit)

I used to ask my clients to limit fruit to 2–4 servings a day, but, as with vegetables, no one ever got fat from eating too much whole fruit. Whole fruits are nutritious and full of fiber and nutrients. Fruits in whole form have so many health benefits that there's no reason to limit them. Whole fruits are nature's dessert—they're sweet, juicy, and delicious and there's no added sugar. Fruits contain fructose, a natural sugar, but because you're eating the whole food—fiber and all—the body takes its own sweet time processing it. As with vegetables, the fiber naturally limits how much fruit you can eat. Most people have a hard time eating more than 3 servings of fruit a day anyway. So do your best to eat the recommended amount and know that it's okay to eat more if you're hungry and fruit looks good to you. But keep it whole!

Keep it whole

Only a fraction of Americans (mostly young children) eat enough fruit, and some of it comes in the form of apple, orange, and other fruit juices,[2] dried fruit, fruit smoothies, or canned fruit. Eating these processed fruits is okay on occasion but has some drawbacks.

Fruit juice doesn't have nearly as much fiber as the whole fruit from which it came. When you drink it, the body absorbs the sugar (fructose) quickly. It's also much easier to overconsume juice. Because it doesn't have the fiber, you just don't fill up on it the same way you do with whole fruit. If you drink fruit juice, stick to 100 percent juice and limit it to 4 ounces a day.

Dried fruit is just what it sounds like: fruit minus its water content. In this concentrated form (1 cup grapes equals ¼ cup raisins), fruit is much higher in sugar and calories. In addition, the portion shrinks considerably when dried, making it easy to overeat.

Fruit smoothies made with juice or more than 1 cup fruit fall into the same category as juice and dried fruit. If you like fruit smoothies, make them at home whenever possible and stick with a 1-cup portion of fruit, milk (or your favorite milk swap) if desired, plus ice. And enjoy a smoothie no more than once a day. When you do buy a smoothie, order the smallest size and steer clear of the giant store-bought smoothies, which are often quart-sized (32 ounces).

Lastly, unless you live on a frozen island with infrequent food deliveries, there's really no reason to turn to canned fruit, especially the ones in sugary syrup.

Life is a bowl of cherries

Need some tips for making fruit a regular part of your day? For variety, choose your fruit according to the season—berries and cherries in spring and summer, grapes and apples in the fall, oranges in the winter. Seasonal fruit is not only fresher but also less expensive than out-of-season items. Another option is to turn on the heat and pump up the flavor by cooking your fruit. Baked apple or pear with cinnamon takes on a whole new dimension. Do the opposite and pair a peeled banana with a schmear of peanut butter, put it in a baggie, and freeze it like a Popsicle! Speaking of Popsicles, you can make a fruit pop by freezing 3–4 ounces of juice, pureed fruit, or a blend of pureed fruit and milk. The perfect healthy treat!

FRUITS AND VEGETABLES ARE NOT THE CAUSE OF OBESITY

Produce has calories, but I guarantee you that no one ever got fat from eating too many vegetables (unless they overdid the butter, oil, or salad dressing) or too much whole fruit (unless it's dried, laden with sugar, or stuffed in a piecrust). And according to the *2015–2020 Dietary Guidelines for Americans* (the nation's go-to source for nutrition advice) and the Centers for Disease Control and Prevention, with few exceptions, Americans do not eat nearly enough of these fresh whole foods.[3] So, I'm giving you permission to eat as many as you want, with just a few key exceptions.

A study conducted by the commercial weight-loss program Weight Watchers found that allowing dieters, even those with diabetes, to eat as many fruits and veggies as they wanted gave them an emotional boost because they didn't feel deprived. The program also offered support, including diabetes education and an online community.[4]

Fruits and veggies offer a boatload of nutrients for the calorie count, so giving you unlimited access to these nutrient-dense gems won't— I repeat, will not—cause weight gain. And because they are packed with fiber, which signals your body to feel full, you can eat only so many of them anyway. When you fill up on fruits and veggies, you tend to eat fewer empty calories.

If you're not accustomed to getting a lot of fiber and suddenly do an about-face and eat a lot of produce, your stomach may initially rebel. So, I suggest you start slowly and work your way up to eating more produce. (Note: Some of you may tolerate cooked veggies better than raw.) I also suggest avoiding cereals and crackers that have 15–20 grams of fiber per serving, as these products will likely give you a stomachache and a bloated belly.

STARCHES (GRAINS AND STARCHY VEGETABLES)

How much?	4–6 servings
What is a serving?	Bread, 1 slice
	Cold cereal (with at least 3 grams of fiber), about 1 cup
	Corn, 1 ear or ½ cup
	Crackers, 1 ounce
	Grain (see whole-grains list), ½ cup cooked
	Legumes (chickpeas, black beans, lentils, split peas, white beans), ½ cup cooked
	Popcorn, 3 cups plain, air popped
	Potato, sweet potato, ½ baked or ½ cup
	Starchy vegetables (see starchy vegetables list), ½ cup unless otherwise noted with an asterisk
	Winter squash (butternut, acorn), 1 cup*
Go for it:	All starchy vegetables and whole grains
Put a lid on it:	Refined grains (white bread, white pasta, white rice), sugar-sweetened cereal

I like to break starches into two groups: grains and starchy vegetables. Starchy vegetables and whole grains are storehouses of fiber and vitamins and minerals, including folate, magnesium, and antioxidants. You can't eat unlimited amounts of them like you can fruits and nonstarchy vegetables—if you eat too many starches, you will eventually feel some love handles. But when you eat healthy starches in thoughtful portion sizes, they can actually help you lose weight. Including a sweet potato, quinoa, or brown rice with your dinner comfortably fills you up, especially when just eating a salad isn't going to cut it.

WHOLE GRAINS

Brown rice	Bulgur (cracked wheat)
Buckwheat flour	Kasha (buckwheat)

Millet	Whole-grain barley
Popcorn	Whole-grain corn / corn meal
Quinoa	Whole oats / oatmeal
Sorghum	Whole rye
Sprouted grains	Whole-wheat flour (bread, pasta, crackers)
Triticale	
Whole farro	Wild rice

STARCHY VEGETABLES

Cassava	Plantains	Sweet potatoes
Corn	Potatoes	Winter squash (butternut, acorn)*
Legumes	Pumpkin	
Parsnips	Rutabagas	

Going against the grain (refined grains)

According to the *Dietary Guidelines*, Americans eat more than enough grains, which is a problem because most people relish the unhealthy variety—or what we call refined grains. Refined grains such as white bread, pasta, and white rice go against the grain when it comes to health and weight loss. Refined grains have been stripped of most of their nutrients (including fiber) through the manufacturing process. Although they are enriched with several B vitamins and iron, refined grains are not nearly as nutritious as whole grains and should be included in your diet sparingly.

Eating refined grains every now and then in small portions is fine, but most Americans eat too much pasta, pizza crust, crackers, cereals, bagels, rolls, muffins, cakes, and cookies made from refined flour. It's easy to do because refined grains are often in grab 'n' go

A KERNEL OF TRUTH

Popcorn kernels are whole grains, making popcorn a great snack for volume lovers—people like my mom, who loves large portions. Three cups of air-popped popcorn (about 1 tablespoon unpopped) is 1 starch serving, compared with ¾ cup of pretzels. Just avoid drenching the fluffy delights in butter.

foods available almost everywhere, from coffee shops to convenience stores to restaurants.

The refined-grain equation isn't good for weight loss. Refined grains contain the same number of calories as whole grains, but their lack of fiber leaves you feeling unsatisfied. I encourage you to limit your intake of refined grains and fill up on this starch's better half: whole grains.

Grist for the mill (whole grains)

Whole grains work for you in your weight-loss efforts: Think of them as grist for the dieter's mill. Like a pile of grain during harvest season, the evidence keeps mounting. According to research from Boston University, consuming whole grains reduces the risk of obesity and weight gain, especially around the waistline. People who ate whole grains had on average smaller waist circumferences than those who ate refined grains or no grains. And you might find it even more interesting that eating at least 3 servings of whole grains a day helps to reduce the risk of chronic diseases—namely, heart disease, type 2 diabetes, and some types of cancers.[5]

On average, Americans get only 1 serving of whole grains a day—maybe a slice of whole-grain toast or oatmeal at breakfast.[6] I know you can do better than that. Add whole-grain cereal to yogurt,

You can tell whether a product is whole grain if the packaging indicates that the food is made from 100 percent whole grains.

The Whole Truth

Don't be fooled by "multigrain," which simply means two or more grains. Some products use a combination of whole grains and refined grains. So check the ingredient list. Unless the ingredient list uses the word "whole" in front of the grain (whole wheat, whole oat, whole rye...), you're probably eating a refined product that has been stripped of fiber as well as some vitamins and minerals during the manufacturing process—and sometimes colored with molasses to make it look like it is made from whole grains.

eat brown rice instead of white, and always choose whole-grain breads.

Man and woman cannot live on whole grains alone. But without them, you're missing some key protective factors—and some delicious foods.

Starchy vegetables

I gave you a list of starchy vegetables on page 29. We set these vegetables apart from the freebie varieties because starchy vegetables have more carbohydrates and calories than nonstarchy vegetables. This scares a lot of dieters away. But when eaten in thoughtful portion sizes—and prepared healthfully—starchy vegetables are perfectly fine to enjoy on the Plan. Just as with grains, you'll get fat from eating starchy vegetables only if you eat too much or smother them with lots of oil or sauce.

Take baked potatoes. Like other starchy vegetables, baked potatoes are high in fiber, which fills you up and aids in digestion. They contain potassium, vitamin C, magnesium, vitamin B6, and folate. French fries, and even sweet potato fries, are another story (unless you *roast* a healthy version yourself). When deep-fried, potatoes lose a lot of their nutrients and gain a lot of fat and calories. Because fries don't offer much in the way of nutrition and are really just a source of added calories, they're on the treats and sweets list.

It's all about portion control. I include a sweet potato or a baked potato in my diet on a regular basis and have never gained any weight from them. I stop at one. I do not eat the biggest one in the supermarket (some are huge!), and I watch what I top it with. I drizzle on some olive oil (which is healthier than butter and, to me, tastes better) and that's it. I always skip the sour cream because I see no point in loading up on multiple fats at once. And I stay away from greasy French fries. I do enjoy homemade roasted sweet potato and butternut squash fries, drizzled with a little oil, on occasion. And you can too.

The five rules of starch

Starches are one of the easiest food groups to overdo. Some people can eat a small amount of starch at all three meals. For those of you who have a hard time portioning your starches, I suggest including them in only one or two meals a day, as many of my clients do successfully. When you do eat them and follow these five simple rules, you supercharge your weight-loss plan as well as your health.

Eat it all! Eat the whole grain, that is. I cannot emphasize this enough. Take advantage of the health perks of whole grains—not to mention the flavor and fullness factors. Refined grains not only lack these benefits but, when eaten in excess, may lead to the diseases that whole grains protect against.[7]

Get the real McCoy. Look for the word "whole" as a first ingredient. The major ingredient in refined white bread, for example, is enriched wheat flour. *Enriched* does not mean better than whole. Food producers must enrich white bread with nutrients that are lost in the milling process. Whole grains are far more nutritious.

Give me some skin. Whenever possible, eat the jackets. Keep the skin on starchy vegetables such as potatoes and sweet potatoes when you cook and eat them. The skin is loaded with fiber, vitamins, and other nutrients. It tastes good too.

Make it steamy. Preparing your starchy vegetables by either steaming, roasting, baking, microwaving, or sautéing them with a drizzle of extra-virgin olive oil is healthy and delicious. Avoid boiling them, however. All vegetables lose nutrients to the water when boiled, which is fine if you're making soup, as the nutrients become part of the broth. Otherwise, don't throw out the baby with the bathwater.

Choose thoughtful portions. Watch your starch portions and you will not gain weight from them. There's no need to eliminate them from your diet completely.

LEGUMES: MEAT ALTERNATIVE OR STARCHY VEGETABLE?

I mentioned that the Plan is flexible. Here's a case in point: You can place legumes, one of nature's most nutrient-dense foods, into the starches group or the fish, poultry, meat, and meat alternatives food group. You may know legumes as beans and peas: lentils, green peas, chickpeas, and navy, black, and kidney beans, to name just a few. Legumes are a staple for vegetarians and those cutting back on animal sources of protein. Hence, the option. And, to put the icing on the cake (or the hummus on the cracker), you can alter which food group you place legumes in to suit your daily whim.

FISH, POULTRY, MEAT, AND MEAT ALTERNATIVES

How much?	2–3 servings (6–9 ounces)
What is a serving?	3–4 ounces of fish, poultry, meat (beef, lamb, and veal), veggie/bean burger
Meat alternatives:	Hummus, ½ cup
	Legumes (beans, split peas, or lentils), 1 cup cooked
	Tofu, tempeh, 1 cup
	Whole eggs, 2–3; egg whites, 4–6; egg substitute, ½ cup
Go for it:	Fish, skinless poultry, legumes, tempeh, eggs, veggie/bean burger, lean and extra-lean cuts of meat (beef, lamb, and veal) (USDA Select or Choice grades, trimmed, such as round, sirloin, tenderloin, and flank steak)
Put a lid on it:	Bacon, high-fat cuts of meat (beef, lamb, and veal); hot dogs, processed sandwich meats, spareribs, soy burgers (made from processed soy), vegetarian hot dogs

(Note: The protein in 1 ounce of meat, fish, or poultry is equal to the protein in 1 egg, 2 egg whites, or ½ cup cooked legumes.)

This food group is all about protein, protein, protein. The workhorse of nutrients, protein builds muscle and keeps your hair and nails strong and your brain humming. Every one of your body's organs requires it to function. But aside from being the body's building block, protein fills you up and keeps sugar cravings at bay. Most of my clients love hearing that. However, you do not have to eat an entire cow to get your protein or to feel full. It is very easy to overeat this food group, especially if you are going out to your favorite steakhouse, where a rib eye coming in at 16 or 20 ounces contains more than two days' worth of protein.

If you know you're going out to dinner and will likely order fish, chicken, or beef as a main course, I suggest going meatless for lunch and opting for vegetarian protein sources instead—a lentil salad or bean soup with your favorite whole grain, for instance. At the restaurant, be mindful of eating enough veggies so you eat only a portion (your portion) of the cow.

Fish, poultry, meat, and meat alternatives are also rich in vitamins and minerals, including niacin, vitamin B6, iron, and zinc. The best sources of protein are lean: all types of fish, skinless chicken and turkey, and lean cuts of beef such as sirloin or top round roast. When you opt for whitefish or white-meat chicken or turkey, it's okay to give yourself an extra ounce or two on occasion. Aim to prepare different varieties of fish at least twice a week. Fatty fish, including salmon and tuna, is rich in heart-healthy omega-3 fatty acids. Do be mindful of how much red meat you eat; when consumed in excess, it has been linked to cardiovascular disease.[8] I recommend consuming red meat no more than once or twice a week. Consider how you prepare your protein. Choose to grill, broil, poach, or bake instead of fry.

Legumes (lentils, peas, and beans) are high in protein, low in fat, and full of fiber. These meat alternatives keep you full and energized. And, no, they are not fattening when eaten in the right portions. Other meat alternatives include eggs, tempeh, tofu, and edamame. If you're a vegetarian, legumes and soy-based meat alternatives are your go-to proteins, although I suggest skipping the highly processed soy burgers and veggie dogs. If you don't regularly eat legumes, try adding these filling and supernutritious plant-based proteins to your diet to get more bang for your buck when it comes to nutrients and fiber. Take the ½-cup challenge: Challenge yourself to eat at least ½ cup of legumes at least several times a week. Or schedule a meatless Monday to try new vegetarian foods. Who knows? You may want to go meatless on Thursday, too!

DAIRY

How much?	2–3 servings
What is a serving?	Cheese, 1½–2 ounces (2 slices, ⅓ cup shredded cheese)
	Cottage cheese, pot cheese, ricotta cheese, ½ cup
	Milk, milk swaps (almond milk, cashew milk, coconut milk, oat milk, peanut milk, soy milk), kefir, 1 cup
	Yogurt, 6–8 ounces
Go for it:	Low-fat, part-skim, and fat-free dairy; unsweetened milk swaps (calcium- and vitamin D–fortified)
Put a lid on it:	Whole-milk products and sugar-sweetened milks, sweetened milk swaps

Not everyone tolerates dairy. If you don't, I list some options for you in this section. If you do, I encourage you to eat and drink it, as it's a great source of calcium and protein. And, according to the *Dietary Guidelines*, unless you're a toddler, you are likely not consuming enough dairy,[9] so I'm going to milk this section for all it's worth. Having a low-fat Greek yogurt (loaded with protein) at breakfast or a piece of cheese for a snack helps tide you over. Dairy is also packed with essential nutrients, including calcium, potassium, and vitamin B12. Like grains, low-fat dairy has been shown to reduce the risk of chronic diseases, including heart disease and high blood pressure. Dairy's big claim to fame is bone health. Milk, cheese, yogurt, and kefir are rich in calcium, a mineral needed to keep your bones and those pearly whites nice and strong.

So now the big question: full fat or low fat? Lately, there's been much debate over whether full-fat dairy is good for you. I like to tell clients to choose low-fat dairy products most of the time. Full-fat dairy is high in calories but also saturated fat, which, when eaten in excess, has been shown to contribute to cardiovascular disease. Unless leading guidelines in this country, including the *Dietary*

Guidelines[10] and those put out by the American Heart Association,[11] change their position regarding saturated fat, I've no reason to change mine. So with dairy fat, go low most of the time. Low-fat versions are just fine, if you don't like fat-free milk or yogurt.

If you don't like or can't tolerate dairy or are a vegan, choose a calcium- and vitamin D–fortified dairy substitute such as unsweetened almond, cashew, or soy milk. And when opting for nut milks, be aware that you won't be getting much protein. You can eat healthfully without including dairy in your diet. However, it's important that you eat a varied diet of calcium-rich food sources including greens, broccoli, canned salmon and sardines with bones, and almonds.

About now, you're probably wondering whether ice cream, frozen yogurt, and other frozen treats fall within the dairy category. Although some are made from dairy products and have calcium, frozen desserts also have a lot of added sugar, so you can find them in the treats and sweets section.

FATS

How much?	2–3 servings
What is a serving?	Avocado, ¼ cup (¼–⅓ avocado, depending on size)
	Butter, cream cheese, mayonnaise, nut butters, oils, tahini paste, 1 tablespoon (3 teaspoons)
	Coconut, ¼ cup shredded, unsweetened
	Cream, half-and-half, 2 tablespoons
	Nuts, seeds, ¼ cup
	Olives, 12–15
	Salad dressing, 2 tablespoons
Go for it:	Extra-virgin olive (EVOO), grape-seed, canola, and most vegetable oils; olive oil–based salad dressing, tahini, avocado, nuts, nut butters, seeds, olives
Put a lid on it:	Margarine, butter, cream cheese, mayonnaise, creamy salad dressing, tropical oils (coconut, palm kernel, palm)

You might not think of fat as your friend, but it's certainly not the enemy some dieters once made it out to be. Fat is filling and flavorful, and some fats are a good source of vitamin E and essential fatty acids. The body doesn't produce the essential fatty acids on its own yet needs them to maintain optimum health, which means you need to get them from your diet or from a supplement. It's easy to get these healthy fats from foods such as salmon, tuna, flaxseeds, and walnuts, so turn to food over supplements.

Fats also help the body absorb the fat-soluble vitamins—A, D, E, and K. So you might like what I have to say here: Adding healthy fats to your diet in thoughtful portion sizes is necessary for good health.

Like with any food group, you're working with healthy and unhealthy choices. You want to pick the healthiest options and shy away from those that do more harm than good. And you want to always be on portion patrol—which means making sure you add enough (but not too much) healthy fat to your diet. Fats have more calories than carbs and protein (9 versus 4 calories per gram), so put the brakes on how much you use. Added fat comes in many forms: oils, solid fats, and nuts and nut butters, as well as salad dressings, olives, avocados, and condiments such as mayonnaise.

A slippery slope

Most of us use fat in the form of oils (extra-virgin olive oil, canola oil, and sunflower oil, among others) and solid fats (butter, coconut oil) for cooking or moistening and adding flavor to foods. In terms of weight loss, the type of fat you use might not make much difference, but in terms of nutrition and heart health, it pays to know the differences.

All fats are made up of three types of fatty acids—polyunsaturated, monounsaturated, and saturated. Choose unsaturated (poly- and mono-) fat for health and limit saturated fats, which are known to clog arteries. Most oils—the liquid fats—have far less saturated fat than their solid counterparts, including butter and coconut oil. And liquid fats are the fats I recommend using.

You might have noticed that what has become the fat of choice for many—coconut—is under "Put a lid on it." There's a reason for this: The final verdict on coconut oil is not yet out. Most of the current research still claims that saturated fat clogs your arteries, which can ultimately lead to heart disease. And coconut oil, I'm sorry to say, is close to 90 percent saturated fat, which is far more than butter, which comes in at just under 70 percent. Other tropical oils, including palm oil and palm kernel oil, are also high in saturated fat. (Note: Although tropical oils are referred to as oils, they are technically solid fats.)

You can still enjoy some coconut oil in the right portions—and on your hair and skin. Just know that coconut oil is not healthier than a liquid oil such as extra-virgin olive oil. I love coconut and enjoy it in small portions on occasion. But I also don't eat red meat, butter, and most fried foods.

In a 2016 *New York Times* survey, 72 percent of the public (and 37 percent of nutrition experts) considered coconut oil to be healthy.[12]

Does Coconut Oil Accelerate Metabolism or Clog Arteries?

Coconut oil has gotten a lot of press as a fat that can increase metabolism and good cholesterol as well as encourage weight loss. But coconut oil is high in saturated fat. So, is it good or bad for you?

Coconut oil became a superfood when some people misinterpreted a single study conducted by Dr. Marie St-Onge at Columbia University that looked at the effect of medium-chain triglyceride oil (MCT oil) in the body.[13] Dr. St-Onge's study used a special coconut oil made up of 100 percent MCTs, a version not available to the public. The typical coconut oil available to consumers contains just 13 percent MCTs. The special MCT oil, not consumer coconut or MCT oil, aided in weight loss. For the coconut oil you find on the shelf to help with metabolism, you'd have to consume at least 10 tablespoons per day (there are about 11 grams of saturated fat per tablespoon, which is close to the upper limit recommended by the American Heart Association). You'd be defeating your purpose by clogging your arteries, and, very possibly, you'd be gaining weight. Furthermore, while coconut oil is high in the fatty acid lauric acid, which may elevate your "good" cholesterol, it doesn't cancel out coconut's effect on raising "bad" cholesterol.[14]

Be a health nut

Nuts and seeds are a great source of healthy fat, as well as protein and fiber. I place nuts and seeds in the fat group because most of their calories come from fat. They're filling and nutritious but also easy to overeat. To avoid overdoing it, portion out a palm's worth of nuts or seeds instead of eating them out of the bowl (or bag!), and opt for the salt-free varieties. You'll find they are incredibly satisfying.

As nutty as it may sound, regular consumption of nuts is not associated with weight gain.[15] When eaten regularly in thoughtful portion sizes, nuts might even help you shed pounds.[16] When you eat nuts as a snack, you tend to skip the fattening junk food and also eat fewer calories later in the day. Nuts also help to stabilize blood sugar and are good for heart health.

Nut butters, including peanut, cashew, and almond, are also healthy choices. But like nuts and seeds, these spreads need to be portion controlled, as the calories add up quickly.

I will never ask you to count fat grams (or any other grams, for that matter). If you choose healthy portion sizes, you'll be well within the recommended limits. When you sauté vegetables, top your salad with dressing, and make a PB&J, you're the boss when it comes to how much fat you add. So stick to the 2–3 servings of added oils, nuts, and other fats. This translates into 2–3 tablespoons', or 6–9 teaspoons', worth. Fat helps you feel full and does offer health benefits, but if you eat too much, you will likely gain weight.

TREATS AND SWEETS

How much?	0–2 servings

What is a serving?	Alcoholic beverages
	    Beer, 12 ounces
	    Spirits (vodka, whiskey, gin, rum, tequila),
	    1½ ounces
	    Wine, 5–6 ounces

	Cake, 1 ounce (thin slice)
	Candy, ¼ cup
	Chips, ½ cup (10 potato chips; 15 corn chips)
	Cookies, 2 (each 2 inches wide; about 1 ounce)
	French fries, fried onion rings, ½ cup
	Frozen treat (ice cream, sorbet, frozen yogurt), ½ cup, or 1 Popsicle (frozen fruit or fudge pop)
	Pie, small slice, ⅓ cup
	Sugar, honey, maple syrup, jelly, gravies, and sauces, 1–2 tablespoons
Go for it:	Plan for a treat and enjoy it on occasion. Eat only what you love. Don't waste calories on junk food just because it is there!
Put a lid on it:	French fries, big bags or containers of anything, oversized beverages (except water, sparkling water, or herbal tea)

If you have a sweet tooth, chances are good that by following this program, some—or even all—of your sugar cravings will diminish. Including fiber-rich fruits and vegetables, adequate protein, and healthy fats and choosing healthy snacks can curb sugar cravings.

It's kind of like a hidden bonus. Still, every now and then, you might just want to indulge in a favorite treat.

Treats are allowed on this program but not required. So if you're not a big fan of sugary or salty treats, you certainly don't need to start eating them now. The foods in this group are not nutrient dense and therefore give you little in the way of nutrition. But "legalizing" a treat can help you stick to your plan. So when a treat sounds like just the ticket, go for it—but stick to your portions. Research shows that the bigger the container, the more we eat or drink. So, one of the best ways to adhere to the portion-control aspect of treats and sweets is to purchase your goodies in single servings—a bar of ice cream or even a glass of wine. Or buy a big bag or box and portion it out into single servings at home.

Treats and sweets include not only cakes, cookies, ice cream, and chips, but French fries, gravies and sauces, and alcoholic beverages. French fries are made from potatoes, and potatoes are part of the starches group. They're also one of our nation's most popular vegetables. (If I could, I'd add a smiley face here.) But because they really soak up the oil and lose most of their nutritional value when fried, they're really more like a treat. If you can do without them, great. If you must indulge, it's okay. But by all means avoid nibbling the fries off your child's plate. Nibbling can cause weight gain because you most likely don't even know how much you are eating—which means you can easily overeat. And stealing your treat reeks of deprivation, so you might as well order a small portion and enjoy. The same goes for gravies and sauces, which are hidden sources of calories. Keep them to a minimum.

Natural sweeteners such as pure maple syrup, honey, coconut sugar, and molasses are sometimes touted as health foods because they contain some antioxidants and other nutrients. But like white table sugar, these healthy-sounding sweeteners are concentrated and quickly spike blood sugar levels. So these natural wonders are on the limit list as well. If you want to boost your intake of antioxidants, feast on your favorite fruits instead. Or toss your favorite fruit into the freezer and eat it like candy. Frozen blueberries, grapes, melon—you name it—quench your thirst and your sugar cravings.

Alcohol is also a treat, and if you have a glass of wine or a bottle of beer, drink it with a meal. Alcohol can reduce your inhibition and lead you to mindlessly grab chips, nuts, or other munchies. Consuming alcohol with a meal can also prevent a hangover. Skip the oversized glass of wine and 16- or 24-ounce can of beer (yes, they exist!). These jumbo sizes are more like 2–3 servings. When it comes to coffee drinks, keep elaborateness and portion size in mind. Don't do the jumbo-sized (even if it's labeled as small) sweetened creamy drinks—the ones that camouflage the taste of your coffee. Try herbal iced tea or sparkling water instead of soda.

Avoid a binge-food bonanza

Some of you might feel a kindred spirit with certain binge foods, or foods that you tend to overeat, such as ice cream or chips. If that describes you, leave those foods at the grocery store. There's no good reason to keep them on hand when you're trying to lose weight. You could, on occasion, indulge in those treats when you are out with family and friends. Otherwise, make sure to have fresh or frozen fruit around. If you feel a sugar craving coming on, the natural sugar in the fruit will quickly satisfy it. Frozen grapes, for example, are yummy—one of my faves. And frozen blueberries warmed up in the microwave taste just like the filling in blueberry pie (okay, *almost*). Another option is to use protein as a shield against sugar cravings. Scoop out a handful of nuts or seeds and munch on those. Craving salt? Go for air-popped popcorn with a sprinkle of Parmesan cheese or try whole-grain crackers.

Treats and sweets are fun and yummy, and every now and then it just feels good to have one. So when you do have one, plan for it and savor it. Sit down and give it all your attention. Don't eat it on the fly, but make it a guilt-free pleasure. If you stick to your portions, it's guilt-free by default.

The skinny on soda

Soda and other sugary drinks are not on the treats and sweets list. I can't think of one good reason to drink them. Soda, sweetened iced tea, and energy drinks are purely empty calories. And they go really well with fattening snacks. Hundreds of studies have linked sugary sweetened beverages with obesity. Why bother with them? If you feel you're addicted to them, try replacing them with water, sparkling water, or vegetable juice. If you drink more than one sugary beverage a day, cut back gradually if going cold turkey is too hard. See Day #20: Sip Your Way to Slim (page 182) for more ways to cut down on soda.

Finally Full, Finally Slim is a package deal that includes not only healthy foods but water, exercise, and overall self-care as well.

A Package Deal

Moving your body not only burns calories but boosts your mood and leaves you feeling good about yourself. Plan to exercise four to five days a week for at least 30–45 minutes. Water flushes your cells of toxins, helping to keep them clean and pure. It also lubricates your joints and gives your skin a healthy glow. I recommend drinking about 64 ounces of water a day. To keep track of your water intake, use a drinking bottle with measurement lines at first. Herbal teas and sparkling water (with no added sugars or artificial flavors) are also great choices.

Portion control is like a classic wardrobe: It never goes out of style. It's not a trendy fad but a proven method for healthful living.

When you enjoy balanced meals and nutritious foods in appropriate portion sizes, you can get off the weight-loss merry-go-round. So go ahead and enjoy a glass of wine or an occasional ice cream cone (a single scoop!). Eat brown rice, quinoa, and other healthy carbs. It's not only okay. It's the best way to achieve long-term weight loss and maintenance.

STAGE 1
Your Mind-Set

DAY **1** Adopt a New Attitude

DAY **2** Write It before You Bite It

DAY **3** Decode Food Labels

DAY **4** Debunk Health Halos

DAY **5** Eat Food, Not Nutrients

DAY **6** Get Over Your Fear of Carbs

DAY **7** Let Your Hand Lead the Way

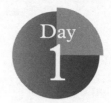

Adopt a New Attitude

> Once you surrender to your vision,
> success begins to chase you.
>
> —Robin Sharma

The first hurdle many of my clients face before they truly commit to losing weight is the fear of failure. *I've failed every diet so far, so why should Dr. Young's program make a difference?* These smart, successful, and insightful people have tried diets before, and they lost weight but didn't manage to keep it off. The reason they regained their weight was because they never learned how to right-size their portions, not because they failed.

If you have a long list of dieting failures, think of each of them as getting you one step closer to this realistic, doable, and healthy program, where food is part of your everyday life. Let every failure go. Whatever you did before, whatever diet you tried, is in the past.

Slice of Advice

Many people lose more inches than pounds, so a true measure of weight loss is not always the scale but your clothes. Periodically try on a piece of tight-fitting clothing you can no longer get into. When your skinny clothes start fitting, that's a true measure of weight loss.

Get real about your goals

When clients ask me how much weight they should lose, I might give them a weight range, but I never give them an exact number of pounds to lose. That just sets people up for failure. Let's say you decide you want to lose 10 pounds this month. You modify your portions and eat healthfully. At the end of the month, you're 3 pounds shy of your goal. You think you've failed, when actually you've changed your habits and lost weight in the process. I'd call that a success, wouldn't you?

You can give yourself a weight-loss goal—as long as it's reasonable and realistic. If you have only 10 pounds to lose, it's reasonable to set a goal of losing 5 pounds in a month. If you're 50 pounds overweight, a loss of 10 pounds or more over thirty days may be appropriate. If you're not sure about what goal to set, ask your doctor. Or do what I often recommend to clients—forget about a magic number of pounds and focus on only one thing: that the number on the scale is going down. As long as you see that number dropping, bringing you closer to a comfortable weight, you are succeeding. And know that weight loss is about more than numbers. It's about looking and feeling great and being able to maintain a healthy weight.

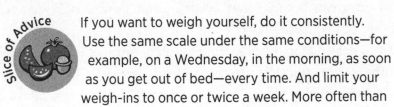 If you want to weigh yourself, do it consistently. Use the same scale under the same conditions—for example, on a Wednesday, in the morning, as soon as you get out of bed—every time. And limit your weigh-ins to once or twice a week. More often than that and you'll be distracted (and worried) by normal weight fluctuations.

Fire it up with some passion

When you want to lose weight, you almost always have a number in mind. That's not really your goal, though. Think about it. *Why* do you want to weigh that specific number? When you manufacture a magic number, what you're really doing is imagining *what your life will be like* at that number. You don't want to get down to a size 6 just for the sake of being a size 6. You want to experience what life is like at that number—what it's like to feel healthier, freer, lighter, more connected, more attractive, and more energetic. And what you want your life to look like stems from your passion.

Passion comes to us for many reasons. Needing to lose weight for a health condition can bring serious motivation. But the desire to effortlessly button up your jeans is reason enough. Now is the time to use your passion to your advantage.

If you feel you need to fire up the passion, visualize yourself at your perfect weight. Every day. I personally believe that it is helpful to visualize yourself doing anything before you actually do it. It's been proven: *The brain can't distinguish between reality and imagination.*[1] If you imagine, really *feel*, what it's like to be or do something, the brain believes it is so. Neurons start firing left and right, waking up your subconscious mind to come up with creative ways to reach your goal. Motivation and passion build and inspire you to take action.

Slice of Advice

Take a 5-minute visualization break every day and picture yourself at your ideal and comfortable weight. What are you doing? How are you dressed? Are you happy, energetic? Does your stomach feel flat? Engage your senses so you *feel* it. And keep it positive.

Make it legit: Commit

When passion and commitment join forces, watch out! Commitment is where you drop excuses and fear and go for it. It's when you decide to put your passion into action. Commitment doesn't mean being rigid and superhard on yourself. I like to think of it happening gently and with self-compassion, such as when you simply "surrender to your vision."

If you don't feel committed, ask yourself what is holding you back. Is it fear of failure? Fear of success? It's usually fear of something. But rather than take you through years of therapy, I'm going to give you some easy advice: What you resist persists. In other words, the more you resist doing something, the more the universe is telling you to do it. Plow through the resistance. Bulldoze if need be. There's a rainbow on the other end.

Gratitude *is* the attitude

I love quotes. In fact, I start most days reading an inspirational quote. It helps me set the stage for a great day. Then at some point, either sometime over the course of the day or before calling it a night, I write down five things I'm grateful for. It's not always a fresh list—sometimes there's some repetition throughout the week. But I'm truly grateful for these things, and writing them down makes me happy. If I've had a bad day, everything changes. Any negativity I'm carrying around magically transforms into gratitude.

I recommend keeping a gratitude journal. It is the fastest, easiest, most effective way I know to improve an attitude. According to a number of gratitude researchers, the benefits cross all areas of life, from relationships to quality of sleep to reduced stress and improved self-esteem. According to University of Illinois researchers, being grateful also keeps you healthier than those who focus on the negative, partly because when you feel positive, you're more likely to do positive things such as work out and schedule your annual checkups.[2]

Thinking of things to be grateful for is easy. Are you breathing? Do you have a roof over your head? A bed to sleep on? Sometimes the little things are the most gratitude-worthy—the hot cup of coffee in your hand, the smile you receive from a passerby, the sound of birds chirping in the early morning hours. The more you realize what you have to be grateful for, the more grateful you naturally become. And life suddenly looks better than ever. So why not open up the doors to receiving more of the good things in life? Open them wide! Start by being grateful you have healthy foods to eat, the desire to be the best you possible, and the knowledge you need to get started. Acknowledging what you're grateful for opens you up to receiving more of the good things in life—including the body and weight you want for yourself. And you don't have to do it all alone.

Take advantage of the buddy system

Instead of tackling weight loss on your own, get a support system going. Researchers from Stanford University learned that good, supportive company can help you ditch excess pounds. In the study, 72 percent of overweight or obese women with a good support system lost weight, compared to only 46 percent of those who didn't call in the troops.[3]

Having at least one other person in your corner helps keep you accountable and encourages you when you need it most. This includes your workouts. If you prefer classes at a yoga studio or fitness center, make a plan to meet one of your pals there. You're more likely to show up, and your workout becomes a fun and friendly social opportunity to boot.

By the same token, skip lunch dates with your fast-food pals. Spend time with them doing something that doesn't involve food so you don't get sucked into old habits. The people you hang out with may affect your weight and your health. Your buddies influence what you perceive to be normal. If the people you surround yourself with are overweight, and you start putting on weight, you're more likely to go with the flow.[4] It's like the old saying—if you hang out in a barbershop long enough, you'll get a haircut. Surround yourself with positive and encouraging like-minded people. They will help you reach your goals.

Bite-Sized Goodie Being optimistic does more than brighten your outlook. It also leads to healthier eating. Researchers who investigated the relationship between optimism and diet quality in postmenopausal women enrolled in the Women's Health Initiative found that the optimistic women were three times more likely to eat healthier than the Debbie Downers in the group.[5]

Believe in yourself

It helps to believe that you can do something before you try to do it. If you don't truly believe you can lose weight, don't worry—you can change your beliefs by changing your thoughts. Saying daily affirmations has been shown to improve health, reduce stress, and boost achievement.[6] Every morning, when you get up, repeat some simple affirmations to help you build that self-belief. A daily affirmation is like a vitamin for the mind. You might want to try saying some of the following:

"I can lose weight—and keep it off."
"I can do it. I'm in control."
"I'm taking it one day at a time."
"Today is the only day that matters."
"The past is the past."
"Every day, I'm making good choices."
"I'm proud of my progress."
"I know what to do, and I am doing it."
"I accept myself and my body and look at the beauty of who I am."

"I am letting go of behaviors that are not healthy."

"I feel good about me."

"I am hopeful that I can do it."

"I am grateful for my body and for getting started now."

"I am influenced by my own decisions—not those of others."

Jot down several statements that resonate with you, put them on a sticky note on your bathroom mirror, and say them every morning while you're getting ready for your day. Your belief in yourself is like a muscle. Develop it and it will get stronger over time. Before you know it, success will be chasing you.

Wedge of Wisdom

When Marni, a thirty-five-year-old lawyer, came to see me, she wanted to lose 30 pounds. She was skeptical and negative and talked about how difficult other diet plans had been for her. She tended to look at the glass as half-empty rather than half-full. Marni and I talked about food. Then we talked about positive thinking. (I guess you could call me a nutritionist and a food shrink.) I asked Marni to keep a food journal and a gratitude journal, which she did. A month later, she seemed more positive and had lost 8 pounds. When she reached her goal of a 30-pound loss, she was so grateful she sent me a wonderful thank-you card.

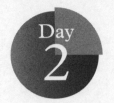

Write It before You Bite It

Three things cannot be long hidden: the sun, the moon, and the truth.

—Buddha

No one wants to be caught with their hand in the cookie jar. And that's why, when it comes to weight loss, the pen (or your favorite app) is mightier than that piece of leftover birthday cake in your refrigerator. Keeping track of what you eat and drink in a journal, notepad, or food-tracking app helps you lose weight—twice as much as those who don't record this insightful information.[1] Studies have shown it to be true. And it will work for you.

How can something so unrelated to food and exercise contribute to weight loss? It keeps you honest. *If you don't write it down, it's almost as if it never happened.* And if you have to write something like "a double-scoop mint chocolate chip ice cream cone," you're more likely to think twice before indulging. Recording what and how much you eat raises your awareness. You see, for instance, how large or small your typical portion sizes are. You might think you eat healthfully but then discover you had only one piece of fruit today and far too many grains. It reveals those truths we would rather overlook. This knowledge helps you make smart decisions about what you will or won't eat for the rest of the day.

Did you mindlessly pick at the roast chicken as you were slicing it? Take a few taste tests of some mashed potatoes? Nibble on your kid's macaroni and cheese? Grab too many appetizers from that party buffet? You might have just forgotten about these nibbles—a case of temporary amnesia. In your heart, you might believe those little cheats don't really count. But they add up. Quickly. If you record them, they suddenly seem more significant.

A food diary gives you a good visual of your food habits. Are you a "see food" eater? Do you eat just because the food is in front of you? This is easy to do at the office, when a colleague brings in free munchies and everyone around you is enjoying the food and cama- raderie. Are you an emotional or a stress eater? Or maybe you're the one who shows up at a restaurant famished and eats the bread basket.

A food diary is so effective that even if it's all you do to lose weight, it will make a difference simply by exposing some of your hidden dietary habits and helping you realize how much you're eat- ing. Recording your intake is one of the best behavior-modification tools ever, partly because it's a painless way to break what I like to call perception deception—believing that you consume more healthy foods and fewer unhealthy foods than you actually do.

Perception deception

It's human nature to discount aspects of ourselves that don't align with our self-image. We might see ourselves as active, healthy indi- viduals. But in reality, we might not be doing nearly as well as we are in our imagination (not to be confused with the visualization exercise we talked about in Day #1: Adopt a New Attitude, page 51, which is far more intentional).

Please don't take this personally. Everyone is guilty of it in one way or another, yours truly included. A food diary has a remarkable way of broadcasting (over a loudspeaker) how wide the gap is between your perceptions and the truth regarding how much and what food you eat in a day. A food diary also shows you what you're doing right—and encourages you to do more of it. Most, if not all, of my clients are surprised at what their food diaries reveal. And they couldn't be happier that they started this little project of self-reflection—mostly because it helps them see why they haven't been able to lose weight. Most clients also realize they don't eat nearly as many fruits and veggies as they thought they did. And they are always surprised at how big some of their other portions are. They see exactly what they need to modify so that it becomes easy to correct a portion size here and there or swap out a choice now and then. And then they start seeing results. Sometimes for the first time in many, many years.

 Keep it together by adding your gratitude list to each day's diary entry and give yourself a star or checkmark for the days you spend time visualizing the new you.

The perfect trifecta

I highly recommend that you keep a record of your food intake for at least thirty days. After the first few days, it becomes second nature. Yet, as powerful and simple as a food diary is, not everyone has the time or inclination to keep it up for thirty days. So I give you three choices: the food diary, the prediary, or the cheat diary.

The **food diary** is quite simple. You just record a few facts. And be specific:

- What you ate
- How much

- The food group
- How you prepared it

My only other request is that you do it in real time, recording as the day goes along. If you wait until bedtime or the next day, you'll likely have forgotten a thing or two...or three.

You can also record your mood or who you were with if you'd like. Some people notice a pattern of eating more when they are stressed or overtired, for instance, or out with a certain group of friends. If you notice a negative pattern, you can take steps to interrupt it.

The **prediary** works well for you forward thinkers who prefer not to live on the fly. Instead of writing down what you ate, you record what you *will* eat, how much, the food group, and how you will prepare it. This works great for ordering in or dining out, so you don't get swayed by colorful images on the menu or the evening's specials. You may want to keep a prediary on days you eat out or order takeout, regardless of which diary format you normally use. For added reinforcement, send yourself an "e-meal"—email yourself a note on what you plan to eat (and then stick to it!).

Use your prediary to record what you actually ate as well—just use a different colored pen or a different computer font to add or change an item, and place a check mark next to the foods you ate.

The **cheat diary** is for those of you swamped with a demanding job, kids, or travel. If you're supershort on time, at least commit to writing down your cheats, those quick, mindless bites that you lose track of. Jot them down as you go. They're so mindless they're frighteningly hard to remember at the end of the day.

Spend time planning your meals. A national survey of more than one thousand adults revealed that people who planned their meals and engaged in other self-monitoring practices lost more weight—and kept it off—than those who did not plan their meals.[2]

Beware of operator error

As remarkable as this weight-loss tool is, it's not foolproof. Keep an eye out for some of these common operator errors:

- Forgetting to record something
- Not paying attention to or underreporting your portions
- Waiting until the end of the day

And be wary of using apps to track calorie counts. First, you don't have to count calories (remember, I've already done it for you). You just need to count your portions and indicate the food group they belong in, which is far less tedious and far more helpful. Second, many of the calorie-tracking apps are inaccurate. It's impossible for them to count calories with 100 percent accuracy because they have no idea what really goes into your dish or exactly how much you really ate. So save yourself some time and focus on what really counts—your portion size.

 Check out Appendix B (page 259). In addition to thirty mix-and-match portion plans, I provide several complete meal plans with the food groups and number of servings.

Regardless of whether you use the food diary, prediary, or cheat diary, you can easily find journals and apps to help you track your food intake. Feel free to use any format you like; just be sure to record the elements covered in this chapter—especially portion size. While many of the available journals and apps require you to indicate portion size, there's no way to check them off for each food group, *Finally Full, Finally Slim* style. For that reason, you might want to photocopy and use the Portion Tracker I provide on page 285, at least in the beginning. You can always add food groups to the notes section of your favorite app, if you prefer. Use the method you will most likely remember to do.

Using the Portion Tracker is easy:

1. Write down what you eat and drink throughout the day, including your portion size and method of preparation.
2. Indicate the correct food group and number of servings for each entry.
3. Cross off each food group serving (with an X) on the diary corresponding to the correct food group icon. If you ate half a serving, cross off with a slash (/).
4. Check to see that you ate the correct number of servings from each food group to match your plan.
5. Be sure to track water, exercise, daily progress, and daily gratitude.

Sample Portion Tracker

Food (include method of preparation)	Your portion	Food group	Number of servings
BREAKFAST:			
Apple berry oatmeal:			
Oatmeal	1 cup (cooked)	Starch	2
Blueberries	1/2 cup	Fruit	1/2
Apple	1/2	Fruit	1/2
Low-fat milk	1 cup	Dairy	1
Flaxseeds (ground)	1 teaspoon		

Food (include method of preparation)	Your portion	Food group	Number of servings
LUNCH:			
Mixed greens	2 cups	Vegetable	2
Carrots, cucumbers, tomatoes, red peppers (chopped)	1 cup	Vegetable	1
Chickpeas	1/2 cup	Meat alternative	1/2
Hard-boiled egg	1	Meat alternative	1/2
Honey-mustard vinaigrette	1 tablespoon	Fat	1/2
Avocado toast:			
Sprouted whole-grain bread	1 slice (1 ounce)	Starch	1
Avocado	2 tablespoons	Fat	1/2
SNACK:			
Frozen banana:			
Banana	1	Fruit	1
Peanut butter	1-2 teaspoons	Fat	1/2
DINNER:			
Vegetable soup	8-10 ounces	Vegetable	1
Grilled salmon	4 ounces	Fish	1
Olive oil, lemon, spices	1 teaspoon	Fat	1/2
Roasted butternut squash	1 cup	Starch	1
Sautéed broccoli and snap peas	1 cup cooked	Vegetable	2
Sesame oil	1-2 teaspoons	Fat	1/2

Food (include method of preparation)	Your portion	Food group	Number of servings
TREAT (OPTIONAL):			
SNACK:			
Rainbow smoothie:			
Raspberries, blueberries, blackberries	1 cup	Fruit	1
Unsweetened vanilla almond milk (calcium fortified)	1 cup	Dairy	1
Peanut powder	1 tablespoon		
1 cup crushed ice			
Vanilla powder and cinnamon			

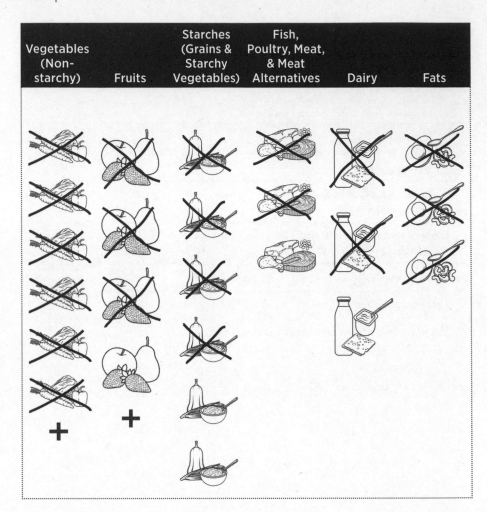

Treats & Sweets:

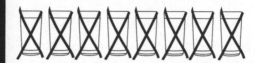

Water:

Exercise:

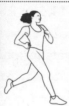

I hour of power yoga

Daily Progress:

Lost 2 pounds since last week! Total weight loss over the last 4 weeks is 7 pounds. Weight this morning was 152. My clothes are starting to get looser around the waist. I'm starting to feel more energized. This plan is agreeing with me. I feel I can keep doing it.

Daily Gratitude:

I'm grateful for my good health.
I'm grateful that I have a job I love.
I'm grateful for my neighbor, who is also a good friend.
I'm grateful I can still drink a cup of coffee on this plan.
I'm grateful I'm losing weight!

Some things in life cannot be denied: The sun sets in the west, what goes up must come down, and recording what you eat and drink shatters perception deception.

Wedge of Wisdom

Rob was what I call a mindless muncher. He had no idea what or how much he ate throughout the day because he rarely sat down long enough to enjoy a meal. A busy hedge fund manager, he was always on the go. He would grab a snack here, a sandwich there, a few forkfuls off his son's plate, or whatever was closest to his fingertips when he felt stressed or hungry. I knew Rob would not take the time to keep food records of everything he ate, so I came up with the cheat diary. Rob recorded all his cheats for only six days, but that's all it took. He went from mindless nibbling to mindful eating and, within a month, lost 15 pounds.

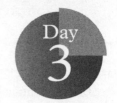

Decode Food Labels

According to serving sizes, I am a family of four.

—Jamie Capria

The FDA requires food and beverage packages to display a Nutrition Facts label, which lists relevant details about the contents, including serving size, number of servings per package, calories, grams of fat, carbohydrates, protein, and other nutrients. The FDA also requires a listing of ingredients in descending order by weight. All of this information can help you decide whether you approve of what you're getting, and it keeps food manufacturers honest about what they're selling you.

The FDA has updated the Nutrition Facts labels on food packages for the first time in about a quarter of a century.[1] I'm not talking about changes in the nutritional content of the foods themselves. I'm referring to changes in the way the content is presented to you, the consumer. Knowing what has changed and how to decode the iconic labels is essential if you want to lose weight, especially because how you interpret the information could skew your idea of how many calories you're consuming. Food companies with $10 million or more in annual food sales must use the new labels by 2020, although many companies have already adopted them.

Before the Nutrition Labeling and Education Act of 1990, which standardized nutrition label serving sizes, food companies were free to determine their own serving sizes. Having similar products with different serving sizes was like comparing apples to oranges when you just wanted to know which brand had fewer calories. One brand of granola might have displayed the calories and nutrients for a ¼-cup serving, while another brand might have used 2 tablespoons. The burden of figuring out which product had more calories was on consumers.

Comparing Apples to Apples

More troublesome was that many companies used the panel as a marketing tool by displaying serving sizes far smaller than any typical person would consume. Because most people ignore the serving size and home in on a product's calorie count, it worked. When new, standardized serving sizes came out in the early nineties, consumers actually complained to manufacturers about the increased number of calories in their foods! They did not realize that it was just the serving size that increased. This time around, the FDA has changed about 20 percent of serving sizes, so don't be surprised if some of your favorite foods now appear to have more (or fewer) calories.

Manufacturers with less than $10 million in annual food sales will have an extra year to comply.

The label makeover

Rising obesity rates, new science, and recent dietary intake survey data about current eating habits (yes, we are eating more than we ate in the past!) contributed to the decision to update the Nutrition Facts label. As a result, the following parts of the label are changing in an effort to help you make more informed choices that support a healthy diet:

Nearly 20 percent of serving sizes have changed—and most of them are bigger. For example, the serving size of ice cream increased from ½ cup to ⅔ cup and soft drinks went from 8 ounces to 12 ounces, while yogurt decreased from 8 ounces to 6 ounces. Go figure…food manufacturers shrunk the size of the yogurt container and, therefore, we eat less of this healthy food!

The font size used for the serving size and number of calories is much larger, so you can finally see this information without a magnifying glass.

"Added sugars" gets its own line. Now you can distinguish between naturally occurring sugars (found in fruit and dairy) and added sugars.

Packaged foods that are generally eaten in one sitting (a small bag of chips, a 20-ounce soda) are labeled as 1 serving. The previous serving size (and servings per container) on a 20-ounce soda bottle, for example, was 8 ounces (and 2½ servings). However, most people don't share a single-serve 20-ounce bottle of soda with 1½ other people.

Food packages that include multiple servings but that some people would typically eat in one sitting (such as a pint of ice cream or a 24-ounce soda) now have a dual-column label—one for the serving size and one for the entire package.

The number of calories from fat is disappearing. It never really told us much.

Manufacturers are required to list the daily value (DV) for vitamin D and potassium because most Americans don't get enough of these nutrients.[2] Note that the DV for vitamins A and C used to be required but is now optional because most Americans get enough of these nutrients. Quick history lesson: The FDA developed DVs to aid consumers in comparing nutrient levels in the food they consume to the daily amounts their bodies require. Since then, labels must include percentage DVs so we can easily see how a serving of food contributes to our total daily need (and lets us know when we've surpassed that need).

Let's look at each of these changes more closely.

Bite-Sized Goodie

To avoid eating more calories than you bargained for, always check the serving size on the food label. A Colorado State University study revealed that, when glancing at Nutrition Facts labels, people pay attention to the calories and nutrient content and often ignore the serving size.[3] In another study conducted by the Center for Science in the Public Interest, 62 percent of consumers ate an entire can of soup (2–3 servings) in one sitting because they assumed it was a single serving.[4] They mistakenly thought they were eating a fraction of the calories they actually consumed.

Serving size: A breach in numbers

The Nutrition Labeling and Education Act requires that serving sizes listed on Nutrition Facts labels reflect *current eating habits*. The serving sizes on the labels, therefore, are based on how much we actually eat, *not necessarily how much we should eat*. The old labels were well behind the times. They were, in fact, published back in 1993 (think: *Sleepless in Seattle*) and based on data collected from surveys taken in the 1970s and 1980s (when a gallon of gas cost 86 cents and Sony Walkmans were all the rage). So the FDA decided it was time for an overhaul.

The agency looked at more recent dietary intake surveys, which reveal that our consumption patterns have, indeed, changed: We are eating more, or less, of close to 20 percent of foods than we were thirty to forty years ago. For example, Americans now consume larger servings of soda, ice cream, and bagels and smaller portions of yogurt. To keep it real, the food label serving sizes are increasing for ice cream, soda, and some bread products; decreasing for yogurt; and staying the same for pizza and burritos. Just to name a few.

Using typical serving sizes is important because the serving size has a domino effect when it comes to the rest of the numbers on the label. A bigger serving size will reflect more calories—along with more sodium, sugar, and other nutrients—on the label. Now when you skim the label on your favorite pint of ice cream, you might notice that the serving size is ⅔ cup instead of ½ cup. Likewise, the number of calories and grams of fat and sugar have also increased. But remember: The FDA is not suggesting that you eat a larger serving of ice cream. The purpose of increasing the serving size is to give you a clear picture of how many calories—and nutrients—you would consume if you did eat a typical serving size.

Do Americans understand food label serving sizes?

The flip side of displaying typical serving sizes on the label is that many people believe that the serving size denotes how much they *should* eat. Note: *Serving sizes on Nutrition Facts labels reflect what people typically eat in a sitting. And since most people eat too much, the serving size on the label is not necessarily the amount you should eat!*

A Georgetown University McDonough School of Business study found that the new labels worked as intended: Participants had a better understanding of how many calories were in a package and ate less of foods they perceived as being unhealthy.[5] A study conducted at New York University's Stern School of Business and Duke University found the opposite of the Georgetown researchers: Most people—nearly 80 percent—thought the serving size on a label was a recommended serving size, or what you should eat, while only 20 percent knew it reflects how much people typically consume. In the same study, people who saw the new labels ate 41 percent more cookies and served nearly 30 percent more cheese crackers to their guests.[6]

Before issuing their final ruling on label content, the FDA established an open comment period to gather input from the public. I recommended that the FDA add the word "typical" before "serving size" or a footnote to clarify that the serving size is based on the amount typically consumed and is not necessarily a recommended portion size. Otherwise, I support the FDA serving size updates and believe that, once the public is educated about the new labels, these changes will lead to better portion awareness.

Making calories pop

The font size of the calorie count has swelled to 22 points—the largest type size on the label—and must appear in bold. Also highlighted via larger type are the number of servings per container and the serving size. The idea is to grab your attention. Even though we track portions instead of calories, in my eyes this is a major improvement over the tiny type used on the old label.

 Did you know that the FDA allows the calories on Nutrition Facts labels to be off by up to 20 percent? Simply put, this means that your favorite 100-calorie snack may actually contain 120 calories. Another case against meticulously counting calories.[7]

What you see is what you get

Food and beverage packages that are typically eaten in one sitting are now labeled as a single serving. Of all the changes to the food labels, this is one of my favorites because you don't have to do the math. What you see is what you get—if you choose to eat or drink it all, that is. But just because the calories are listed for the entire package doesn't mean you're obligated to consume it in one go!

How sweet it is (or isn't)

On packages already sporting the new labels, you might have noticed an additional line for added sugar, which distinguishes between naturally occurring (fruit sugar, milk sugar) and added sugars. This is a sweet move. The *Dietary Guidelines* advocate consuming no more than 10 percent of calories from added sugar—50 grams (around 12 teaspoons) of added sugar a day for a 2,000-calorie diet.[8] If you're trying to lose weight, I recommend you consume less than that amount. (The American Heart Association recommends no more than 6 teaspoons of added sugar for women and 9 teaspoons for men.)[9] The new labels make it delightfully easy for you to do the math for yourself.

Nutrition Facts

8 servings per container

Serving size   2/3 cup (55g)

Amount per serving

Calories   230

	% Daily Value*
Total Fat 8g	**10%**
Saturated Fat 1g	**5%**
Trans Fat 0g	
Cholesterol 0mg	**0%**
Sodium 160mg	**7%**
Total Carbohydrate 37g	**13%**
Dietary Fiber 4g	**14%**
Total Sugars 12g	
Includes 10g Added Sugars	**20%**
Protein 3g	
Vitamin D 2mcg	10%
Calcium 260mg	20%
Iron 8mg	45%
Potassium 235mg	6%

* The % Daily Value (DV) tells you how much a nutrient in a serving of food contributes to a daily diet. 2,000 calories a day is used for general nutrition advice.

Source: Food and Drug Administration

Bite-Sized Goodie

Tired of reading about DVs, calories per serving, grams of fat, and sugars? Eat fresh, whole foods! Fresh fruits and vegetables are not labeled as "fat-free" or "cholesterol-free," even though they are both. These gems don't need to prove their worth.

Once you understand the concept behind the FDA changes, they make perfect sense. And FDA serving sizes aside, you don't have to be confused. You know where to turn for realistic servings. You're holding the source for proper portions in your hands.

Wedge of Wisdom

Rebecca showed me the fitness and calorie-tracking app she'd been keeping for months. She had consistently recorded everything she ate, along with calorie counts, and couldn't understand why she wasn't losing weight on 1,200 calories a day. But when I asked her how *much* she ate, she said she didn't know. Rebecca, like so many of my clients, had it backward. You cannot determine how many calories you eat if you have no idea how big (or small) your portions are! Like so many other clients, Rebecca went with the default serving size, which, in most cases, was smaller than her portions. Once Rebecca learned she was sometimes eating two to four times as many calories as her app was telling her, she began tracking her portions and ultimately lost weight.

Debunk Health Halos

Any cupcake consumed before 9:00 a.m. is technically a muffin.
—A sign in Magnolia Bakery, New York City, summer 2017

Trusted terms such as "low fat," "healthy," "organic," and "all natural" have a certain aura about them. To be good, you order the gluten-free bread at a health food restaurant, reach for the low-fat salad dressing on the grocery store shelf, or grab the organic macaroni and cheese. You think they're healthier than their conventional counterparts. But are they?

In the nutrition field, we use the term "health halo" to describe healthy-sounding claims that lead consumers to perceive foods to be healthier than they are. Health halos can harm weight-loss efforts in two sneaky ways. First, when you think something is healthy, you give yourself permission to eat more of it, and you might even feel virtuous for doing so. Second, some foods with such claims actually have more calories than you might think. Health halos are kind of like calling a cupcake a muffin if you eat it for breakfast.

It's not that food manufacturers are telling you lies. If a product says it's gluten-free or low fat, you can hopefully trust that it is. But the low-fat salad dressing, for instance, might also pack in more sodium, sugar, and calories than the full-fat version. That salad dressing might also have more artificial ingredients. This program doesn't advocate for low-calorie foods at all costs. No one wants to sacrifice flavor *and* quality for nothing.

The other side of this word game is to call out food components that were never in the product to begin with: "no cholesterol," "gluten-free," "no sugar added." These catchphrases can give even junk food instant cachet. Neither potatoes nor salt has cholesterol, which is found only in animal products. Yet some bags of chips boldly display the words "no cholesterol."

Bite-Sized Goodie — University of Toronto researchers looked at more than 3,000 sugar-containing foods and beverages, 630 of them with no- or low-sugar claims. At least half of them still contained excess sugars and many of the products were not actually lower in calories than their "high sugar" counterparts.[1]

All in a name

Here are some of the top health halos to be wary of:

Low fat / reduced fat / fat-free. Researchers at KU Leuven in Belgium found that low-fat labels on junk food led people to eat more of the food, as well as calories, and continue buying the products over the long run, concluding that low-fat products may contribute to obesity.[2] A University of Washington Foster School of Business study singled out guilt as the reason for selecting desserts with healthy-sounding words such as "lite," regardless of calorie count.[3] I'm not advocating that you feel guilty, but if you're going to splurge, it might as well be for the right reasons. Many products labeled with low-fat or similar claims have more artificial ingredients, preservatives, sugar, salt, and calories than the full-fat versions and are certainly no healthier. So be aware and read the labels.

Gluten-free. Products that contain gluten-free substitutes for wheat, such as rice flour, tapioca flour, or corn flour, aren't necessarily any more nutritious than those they're meant to replace, yet somehow "gluten-free" became synonymous with "healthy." Gluten-free products frequently contain more salt, sugar, and calories and less fiber than their gluten counterparts.[4] And they are more expensive to boot! So unless gluten messes with your digestion, save some bread and go for the gluten.

Organic. Nothing shines much brighter than the halo surrounding "organic." University of Michigan researchers found that people perceived organic cookies as having fewer calories than nonorganic cookies, even when the calorie counts on the packages were identical. Participants felt they could eat organic cookies more often and were less inclined to exercise when eating organic.[5] I'm an advocate of clean eating and recommend purchasing organic produce when possible (see Day #12: Think "Whole-istically," page 122). Just know the power the word "organic" might have over you when it comes to packaged products. Organic cookies? Leave them on the shelf.

Zero calories. Don't be fooled by the sweet sound of 0 calories in beverages artificially sweetened with either aspartame, saccharin, acesulfame K, or sucralose. Researchers at the University of Manitoba in Canada reviewed the results of thirty-seven studies that looked at four hundred thousand individuals over a ten-year period. The verdict? Sugar substitutes rarely help with weight loss, and drinking even one artificially sweetened beverage a day has been associated with greater risk of weight gain, obesity, diabetes, and heart disease.[6] We don't know whether the sweeteners are actually causing the weight gain or other variables are at play. Nonetheless, it's unlikely these substitutes help you *lose* weight, and they are not healthy. I suggest skipping them. See Day #20: Sip Your Way to Slim (page 182) for more on diet sodas.

Healthy-sounding product names. Product names that include a healthy-sounding ingredient can be deceiving. Veggie sticks, those airy, straw-like chips made from vegetable powder, don't come close to replacing vegetables. The same concept applies to words such as "sea salt," "coconut sugar," and "honey," all of which should trigger you to read that nutrition label. Even the word "healthy," when used on a package label, is a health halo.

In keeping up with the latest research on fats and to better serve consumers, the FDA is redefining what the term "healthy" means,

Some Healthy Dialogue

at least when it comes to marketing claims. This is relevant to consumers because, when claiming a product is healthy, food marketers must follow FDA guidelines.

Until recently, the *amount*—rather than the *type*—of fat in a product determined in part whether marketers could display the word "healthy" on food packaging. Products low in fat could (and still can) be labeled with the word "healthy," even if they are high in sugar and not exactly healthy (think: fat-free pudding). Meanwhile, truly healthy products high in healthy fats (think: nuts, which are high in unsaturated fats) were by definition disqualified from using the term.

When a manufacturer of nut bars high in *healthy* fats challenged the guidelines, the FDA changed its tune. As of this writing, the guidelines are in the process of being revised, but for now, the FDA is allowing the type of fat a product has—not how much—to determine in part whether the food producer can market the product using the word "healthy."[7]

However, is the word "healthy" useful on a product's label, or does it encourage consumers to eat more? I suspect the latter. As Dr. Marion Nestle, my New York University colleague, food policy expert, and author of numerous award-winning books and the popular blog *Food Politics*, writes, "Health claims on food packages are not about health; they are about marketing."[8]

What you believe can affect your behavior. To my knowledge, no one has ever suffered from heart disease because of a deficiency of alcohol, yet people in a University of California–San Francisco study who believed alcohol is heart-healthy drank on average 47 percent more than people who didn't consider the popular belief.[9]

Healthy chocolate bars have hit the market too. Although they may contain so-called superfoods such as goji berries and biofermented greens, more is not better! If you eat too much, you'll gain weight.

I'm not suggesting that all foods labeled with health claims are unhealthy or will cause weight gain. I am suggesting that you as a buyer beware. Don't make these perceived good-for-you claims an excuse to eat more. Labeling a product "healthy" does not make it healthy. Not labeling a product "healthy" doesn't make it unhealthy. Portion control is far more important than any marketing claim. So put your blinders on when it comes to health halos, read the labels, and stick to the Plan.

Wedge of Wisdom

Caroline couldn't wait to tell me about the amazing coconut deluxe smoothie she had for lunch. She watched as the server cut a whole coconut in half, scooped out the contents (from both halves!) into a blender, and whipped it up with mixed berries, banana, other fruits, and ice. At a session several days later, Caroline asked me how many calories are in an entire coconut. We looked it up: about 1,400. Yikes. Believing coconuts are überhealthy and that the health drink shop she stopped in would serve only healthy foods, Caroline consumed an entire day's worth of calories and about a week's worth of saturated fat all in one drink.

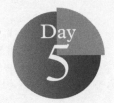

Eat Food, Not Nutrients

A balanced diet is a cookie in each hand.

—Barbara Johnson

If you live long enough, you'll witness the seesaw mentality behind trending diets that focus on one nutrient—namely, fats, carbohydrates, or protein. Current diets have generally divided dieters into two camps. One advocates for a low-carb diet and the other for a low-fat regimen. People can and do lose weight on both of these types of diets. When Dr. Christopher Gardner and colleagues at Stanford University School of Medicine compared the weight loss of people on a low-carb diet with that of people on a low-fat diet in the Diet Intervention Examining the Factors Interacting with Treatment Success (DIETFITS) clinical trial, they discovered that one strategy does not necessarily work better than another for any given person.[1] If you restrict carbs or fats, and eat fewer calories than you burn, you will lose weight.[2]

The bigger, more relevant point is that the majority of people on super-restrictive diets eventually end up regaining their weight. They don't stay on the diet, so it really doesn't matter whether it produces weight loss. What matters is that it doesn't work for them in the long term. In the Stanford University study, the X factor for long-term weight loss was not a single nutrient but the fact that dieters changed their relationship with food. Successful dieters—whether in the low-carb or low-fat camp—were more mindful when eating and ate more meals at home and with family. They changed their behavior and were more satisfied.[3]

Calorie intake, overall food choices, the ability to keep the weight off, and lifestyle—not one nutrient—determine whether any food plan is good for weight loss. When we stop eating an entire food group, we compensate by eating more of something else, and that choice isn't always as healthy as what we're cutting out of our diet. Why not balance our intake of calories across fats, carbohydrates, and proteins by eating healthy food choices from each of the food groups in proper portions? We give ourselves the best chance at long-term weight loss *and* better health.[4]

Bite-Sized Goodie
The *Dietary Guidelines* recommend that your daily food intake be 10–35 percent protein, 45–65 percent carbs, and 20–35 percent fats. But you don't have to do the calculations. I've done them for you. The distribution of nutrients in the Plan falls within these ranges.[5]

The fat-free nineties

The carb-heavy diets of the 1990s are proof in the pudding for how focusing on one nutrient can do more harm than good. The movement to reduce fat in the diet began in the late 1980s, when research linked saturated fats (found in red meat, butter, and full-fat cheese) with heart disease and all fats with weight gain. Many people did their best to limit fat intake, hoping to shed unwanted pounds and get healthy at the same time. So much so that they turned to anything fat-free—big white bagels (served dry, or with no butter) and fat-free muffins the size of bowling balls. In the nineties, even fat-free, sugar-rich treats such as licorice, jelly beans, and candy corn were free for the taking. It's not logical to think that if you eat an entire bag of fat-free licorice you won't gain weight, but I still run into many people who equate *fat-free* with weight loss.

Fat-free dieters made two big blunders. By shunning fat, dieters cut out healthy fats too, such as nuts, nut butters, olive oil, and avocados—all of which are good for you in moderation. Dieters also consumed excess sugar and calories by eating the fat-free cookies and other products that hit the market. (Fat-free processed foods tend to be high in sugar and calories and low in fiber and nutrients.) Instead of losing weight, Americans were putting it on. National dietary intake surveys found that we were eating excess calories—and many of them were coming from carbohydrates.[6] We were inhaling carbs—and not the good ones either.

The pendulum swings

Fast-forward twenty-plus years, and fat is back. Research that condemned added sugar as bad for health, along with new evidence that showed the benefits of good fats, brought fat back and put carbs (especially sugars) on the list of foods to steer clear of. While the Atkins diet, around since the 1970s, has always shunned carbs, some trendy diets (including the keto diet) now focus on eating fats over carbs as a way to trim down. Yet fat has nearly twice as many calories as carbohydrates (9 versus 4 per gram). This puts us right back to where we were in the nineties, just in reverse. We've replaced carbs with fat. Either way, we are eating more calories than we need to and abandoning the health benefits of healthy carbs such as whole grains and starchy vegetables.

Have your cake and eat it too

It's not always about what foods you cut out but what foods you add in. If you eat a handful of nuts with fresh fruit as a snack, there's a good chance you're not going to eat cookies. Fruit and a portion-friendly serving of nuts are all-around healthier choices (containing healthy fats and healthy carbs) for someone looking to lose weight. There are good carbs and good fats. But more is not better. You can't eat as much as you want. Too much of one or the other leads to weight gain. Likewise, if carbs are bad, that alone doesn't make fats good—and vice versa.

Fats are a good example when it comes to singling out nutrients for weight loss or health purposes. All fats have about the same number of calories and can equally contribute to weight gain when consumed in excess. One tablespoon of olive oil has about 120 calories and 1 tablespoon of butter just over 100 calories. "Healthy" fats do not have fewer calories than "unhealthy" fats, so swapping butter (nearly 70 percent saturated fat) for olive oil (about 13 percent saturated fat) is not going to make a difference on the scale. But from a health perspective, olive oil is far better than butter when part of a balanced diet. Olive oil is high in monounsaturated fatty acids (healthy fats). But consuming ½ cup of olive oil a day—or 8 tablespoons' worth and 960 calories—is not going to make us healthier. It would just make us fatter. Always watch your portions, even with healthy foods.

When you take something out of your diet, consider what you're adding back in. Replacing saturated fat (one less-healthy nutrient) with refined carbohydrates (another unhealthy nutrient) doesn't help our cause in the health department. When Harvard researchers compared the risk of heart disease in people with high intakes of healthy fats and whole grains with that in people who ate diets high in saturated fat and refined carbohydrates, they learned that people who ate healthy fats and whole grains had the lowest rates of coronary heart disease.[7]

Bottom line: Focus on eating healthy food in thoughtful portions, not on a single nutrient. Follow the Plan and you can stop worrying about it.

Slice of Advice If you use cooking spray, don't be fooled by all the zeros on the Nutrition Facts label, including the 0 calories and 0 grams of fat. Cooking sprays are mostly fat. But a serving size that contains less than ½ gram of fat can list 0 grams of fat on the label. Increase the serving size and you start to see some numbers. The Nutrition Label serving size for cooking spray is small enough (659 servings in a 7-ounce bottle!) to allow for a label full of zeros. The serving size is also based on a quarter-second spray time, while most people hold the spray button for closer to 6 seconds, which adds up to 50 calories and 6 grams of fat.[8]

Don't let information overload affect how you think about losing weight. You just need to remember two words: portion control. My definition of a healthy diet has withstood the test of time: a wide variety of whole, minimally processed foods from all the food groups in healthy portion sizes. This might not sound sexy, but it works. In *Finally Full, Finally Slim*, we focus on eating food, not single nutrients. No one gets up in the morning and says, *I'm going to eat some saturated fat*. Nor should you.

Likewise, a single food or ingredient doesn't amount to a healthy diet. Organic spinach is healthy. But if that's all you eat, you're setting yourself up for some serious health consequences. Follow the Plan and you won't have to worry about whether fats, carbs, or proteins are good, bad, or indifferent. You won't have to tire of eating a single miracle weight-loss food every day. You just have to make some healthy choices—and enjoy.

Now on to a topic that causes some of you to shudder at the thought of it: carbohydrates.

Wedge of Wisdom

Linda asked if making chocolate pudding with avocados was a good choice for weight loss. When I said no, she was surprised: "But why? It's a healthy fat!" When I replied that healthy foods have calories too, she got the picture. Linda, like many others, acted as if eating healthy fats made the calories disappear.

Get Over Your Fear of Carbs

Every single diet I ever fell off of was because of potatoes and gravy of some sort.

—Dolly Parton

When clients tell me that they've eliminated carbohydrates (aka "carbs") from their diet, my ears perk up. First, I want to know whether our definition of carbohydrates is the same or whether we're using a different lingo. This happens often. When people talk about avoiding carbs, they usually mean starches and sugars. Starches are complex carbohydrates that include grains and starchy vegetables. Sugars are simple carbohydrates. Some are natural (such as fructose in fruit) and some are refined (such as white table sugar).

Once we have word choice squared away, I educate clients about the difference between healthy and unhealthy carbs (aka "carbage"). Some carbs are better for health and weight loss than others. You just need to know which ones. So if you're among the many trendsetters who fear carb-rich foods because you think all carbs lead to weight gain or impede weight loss, it's time to face your fear of carbs—and the facts.

The truth about carbs

Fact #1. Carbohydrates are found in every food group. If you've given up carbs, you've given up food from every food group—as well as all the nutritional benefits that come with those foods. When people tell me they've given up carbs and then proceed to describe the hearty salad and the blueberries they ate for dinner, I kindly explain that if they're eating fruits and vegetables, they haven't given up carbs. In addition to fruits and veggies, foods such as nuts, milk, and legumes all contain carbs.

Fact #2. Healthy carbohydrates can help prevent certain chronic diseases. Carbohydrates found in whole grains contain fiber and an array of vitamins and minerals including magnesium, zinc, manganese, iron, B vitamins, and much more. Consuming healthy portions of whole grains, legumes, and starchy vegetables such as sweet potatoes, along with fruits and nonstarchy vegetables in generous portions, can help prevent common chronic diseases, especially heart disease, certain cancers, and even type 2 diabetes.

Fact #3. Fiber can help with weight loss because it contributes to fullness. Fiber is a dieter's best friend. Fiber, which is found in abundance in *healthy* sources of carbohydrates, is pretty much calorie-free (although the foods containing fiber have calories) and filling. Its goal is to aid digestion and help keep you regular. Fiber also works to maintain healthy cholesterol levels, stabilize blood sugar levels, and protect you from colon cancer. If you're not eating healthy carbohydrates, you're not getting much of any fiber unless you turn to fiber supplements, which I do not recommend.

Throw out the carbage

Let's look at the carbage, or the two unhealthy carbohydrates: refined grains and added sugars.

Refined grains. You may think everyone has given up carbs, but most Americans eat way too many in the form of refined grains—white rice and white bread, cookies, pasta, bagels, pizza crusts, and other items made from refined flour. Eating too many refined grains may increase your risk for heart disease and diabetes, as well as excess abdominal fat.

Choose whole grains over refined grains *whenever possible*. This is easy to do at home, where you're in control of the foods you stock in your kitchen.

Added sugar. The other carbohydrate culprit is *added* sugar, or sugars that do not occur naturally in fruits and milk, for instance. Added sugar has of late been making major headlines. It has been linked to several of the nation's leading killers: heart disease, cancer,

---

People following low-carb diets tend to shun starches altogether, but some starches are good for you. If you follow two simple guidelines, you can enjoy starches and all the benefits that come with them and still lose weight:

Not All Starches Are Created Equal

- Enjoy *whole* grains and starchy vegetables in healthy portions. You won't get fat from eating them *unless you eat too much of them*.
- Avoid or eliminate refined grains, which provide little in the way of nutrition. They've been stripped of the good stuff.

If you want to minimize starches, eliminate refined grains but give the others a fighting chance. When it comes to health and weight loss, whole grains are in your corner.

and dementia. The call to minimize sugar intake is one reason the FDA requires food manufacturers to feature a line for added sugar on the new food label. The average American eats close to 20 teaspoons of added sugar a day—mostly by consuming sodas (a 20-ounce soda has more than 16 teaspoons of sugar!), snacks, and treats.[3]

Added sugars can pile up quickly, especially if we don't even know we're eating them. Hidden sugars are the sugars added to foods we don't tend to think of as sweet—salad dressing, bread, and ketchup, for instance. And a snack that includes 6 ounces of sweetened yogurt and ½ cup of granola can total 29 grams (7¼ teaspoons) of added sugar.

So check the added sugar line on the new food labels and read the ingredients list, which tells it like it is. Reducing added sugars by even a small amount can make a big difference when it comes to weight loss.

Don't confuse naturally occurring sugar with added sugar.

According to the FDA, the nutrient claim "sugar-free" means that a product contains less than ½ gram of sugar per serving. But the term "sugar-free" doesn't mean the product contains fewer calories than the regular version. It may even contain more.

What's the Deal with Sugar-Free Products?

Sugar-free products often contain sugar alcohols such as xylitol, maltitol, or sorbitol. Our bodies don't absorb sugar alcohols very well, so they provide around half of the calories and carbohydrates of sugar. Eating a lot of products made with sugar alcohols can cause stomach discomfort, bloating, and diarrhea. So practice portion control.

My tip: Compare the labels of the regular and sugar-free versions and be sure to check the number of calories as well. And do not have too much of either version. The sugar-free version will probably give you a stomachache if you eat too much.

Fructose in fruit and lactose in dairy are healthy, naturally occurring sugars. While the carton says 1 cup of milk has 12 grams of sugar, it's all natural—not added. Milk also contains protein and calcium, and whole fruit is full of fiber, so you're not going to get that sudden rise in blood sugar when you consume these foods. The sugars in soft drinks, energy drinks, sweetened iced tea, and fruit punch, however, are all added. Nothing natural in those beverages—no fiber, protein, or other components to help your body process the sugar. A food's other components make all the difference.

Carbohydrate weight-gain claims: Fact or fiction?

If carbs have ever been related to weight gain, it's because we like them and so we eat *too much* of them. Size matters! Europe's obesity rates aren't as high as ours, partly because they eat foods in smaller portions. They don't serve 3–4 cups of pasta on a plate. If they do, it's for the entire family. Couple oversized portions with unhealthy refined grains, and you've got double trouble.

People who eat whole grains have, on average, smaller waistlines than people who eat refined grains or *no grains*. Most Americans eat only 1 serving of whole grains a day.[4] The rest are refined. If you're eating the right kinds of grains in the right portions, they don't make you fat. They make you full—and provide you with a battalion of disease-fighting nutrients.[5]

Low-carb weight-loss claims: Fact or fiction?

So many people talk about limiting or banishing carbs from their diet in order to lose weight. They swear by it. So is there any truth to it? The body naturally burns off carbohydrates first, before fat or protein. So the thinking is that if you don't eat carbs, your body will make a beeline for the fat stores and start burning away. But researchers learned another side to the story: People on low-carb diets lose weight not necessarily because they have eliminated carbohydrates but because they tend to eat more whole foods and fewer sodas[6] and, ultimately, fewer calories.[7]

Yale University researchers compared popular diets, from low carb to low fat and low glycemic. When it came to low-carb diets, the resounding verdict was that being *carbohydrate selective* beats being low carb, which reinforces what I've been saying all along: Eat whole grains and starchy vegetables, just eat them in thoughtful portions.[8]

Carbohydrates are so much more than refined grains and added sugars. So I implore you not to demonize all carbohydrate-rich foods because of the processed stuff. Generally speaking, when you cut a food category out of your diet, you tend to compensate by overeating something else, and that's heading into dangerous territory. This kind of extreme behavior leaves you vulnerable to cravings and confusion. Instead of eating the slice of whole-grain toast and a schmear of avocado with your morning eggs, you skip the bread and feel virtuous but not full. To satisfy your hunger, you eat an entire avocado or two, which is far more caloric (even though it's a good fat) and may, indeed, cause weight gain when eaten in excess.

Listen to your body and the facts. Choose nutrient-dense foods from all food groups in healthy portion sizes. You'll feel satisfied. You'll sleep better. You'll be regular. You'll stop obsessing about when you get to eat next. And you'll feel empowered as you fearlessly approach your next meal.

Wedge of Wisdom

Barbara, a very educated and successful author, was cutting out all starches because she couldn't seem to portion control them. She complained that she was always hungry. Together, we took what I like to call the ½-cup challenge: We measured out a ½-cup portion of cooked brown rice and put it on a plate teeming with veggies and a 4-ounce piece of fish. She was more than surprised at how substantial her serving of brown rice looked. And when she ate her starch as part of a balanced meal, she was completely satisfied.

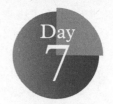

Let Your Hand
Lead the Way

Put your future in good hands—your own.

—Mark Victor Hansen

In my first book, *The Portion Teller Plan*, I introduced a series of visuals readers could use to measure their portions without the aid of any kitchen tools. Visuals are an easy way to eyeball serving sizes and a great alternative to pulling out a measuring cup or food scale every time you eat. Some of the visuals are quite handy—literally, since you use parts of your hand to estimate how much you're about to serve yourself. Others are based on common household items that are easy to instantly produce in the mind, such as a deck of cards.

I have nothing against measuring cups and spoons or food scales. I encourage you to use them early on and at least until you're confident you know how much is on your plate. But for some people, quantifying everything gets old fast. And what happens when you're at a restaurant? You'd probably feel a little foolish whipping out a measuring cup and holding it up to the candlelight to assess whether you're getting a half or a full cup of quinoa.

Portion control should be easy, not stressful, awkward, or interfering. And it need not require perfectionism. Once you get the hang of using visuals and your hand to measure your portions, you'll be guesstimating portion sizes regularly—and doing a good job of it too.

Your portions are in your hands

Your hand is one of the best tools around to help you gauge portion sizes. Not only is it convenient (it's always with you) and made to order (people with big hands can typically eat larger portions that people with small hands), but it works almost as well as using a household measuring instrument. In a University of Sydney study, participants were trained to use the width of their fingers to measure portions, and 80 percent consistently measured within 25 percent of the true weight of the food.[1] Likewise, researchers who evaluated Ireland's food guide found that the palm of the hand was useful for estimating meat portions.[2]

LET YOUR HAND LEAD THE WAY

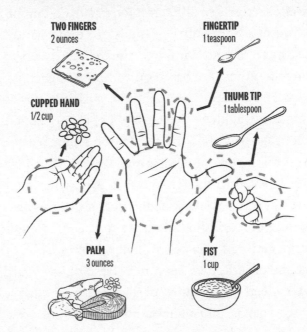

TWO FINGERS
2 ounces

FINGERTIP
1 teaspoon

CUPPED HAND
1/2 cup

THUMB TIP
1 tablespoon

PALM
3 ounces

FIST
1 cup

The hand method is not an exact science, but it does come in, well, handy. Following are some general guidelines for how to be good with your hands by food group. Each example represents a standard unit of measure and not necessarily the amount you should eat of any given food.

Vegetables (Nonstarchy):
At least two cupped hands, *about 1 cup*

Fruits:
Your fist, *about 1 cup*

Starches (Grains and Starchy Vegetables):
Your fist, *about 1 cup*
Your cupped hand, *about ½ cup*

Fish, Poultry, Meat, and Meat Alternatives:
The palm of your hand, *about 3 ounces*
Your whole hand, *about 4 ounces whitefish* (flounder, filet of sole, red snapper)
Your cupped hand, *about ½ cup*

Dairy:
Length and depth of two fingers (cheese), *1½–2 ounces*

Fats:
Layer of your palm (nuts and seeds), *¼ cup*
Knuckle to tip of thumb (oils, nut butters, salad dressings), *1 tablespoon*
Fingertip (oils, nut butter, butter), *1 teaspoon*

Bite-Sized Goodie

Eating healthy portions is not an exact science. It doesn't matter whether you eat 3½ or 4 ounces of meat, for example. You just need to recognize when you've got a 16-ounce steak on your plate and choose to scale back.

Measuring for success

Some people find that common objects make the best ad hoc measuring tools. These visuals are easy to remember. Following are some items you can picture when cooking or eating out.

Baseball—1 cup fruits or vegetables; 1 cup ready-to-eat cereal, cooked pasta, rice, or other cooked grains

Hockey puck—½ cup legumes, hummus, cooked oatmeal or other cooked grains, or tomato sauce

CD case—slice of bread

Computer mouse—1 small sweet potato or baked potato

Checkbook—3–4 ounces whitefish (flounder, filet of sole, red snapper)

Deck of cards—3 ounces salmon, chicken, or meat

4 dice—1 ounce cheese

Cap on a 16-ounce water bottle—1 teaspoon oil, gravy, sugar, or honey

Golf ball—¼ cup nuts or seeds

Shot glass—2 tablespoons oil or salad dressing
½ shot glass—1 tablespoon oil, salad dressing, or gravy

Dental floss container—1 ounce chocolate or a cookie

 Teacup—5 ounces wine

Now put it into action—fill half of your plate with your favorite veggies, a quarter of the plate with healthy protein (1–2 decks of cards), and the other quarter (think one baseball's worth!) with healthy grain such as wild rice, butternut squash, or whole sorghum.

 Here's a little trick I teach clients. This example is for dry cereal, but you can do this with any food: Pour what you think is 1 serving of cereal into a bowl. Before adding any liquid, pour the dry cereal into a measuring cup and see how close your idea of a thoughtful portion is to reality. Chances are, you are giving yourself two or three times more than you might have thought.

The visuals I've introduced you to are fun and easy. Still, I hope you'll take the time to invest in some measuring cups and spoons and a food scale if you don't already have them. (We'll talk more about fun portion props in Day #10: Cook Like a Portion Pro, page 111.) They really can prevent you from derailing your diet by showing you how right or wrong your portion perception has been.

Wedge of Wisdom

Charlie wasn't much of a cook and found it tiresome to measure his food regularly. He also felt as if standard portion sizes were too small for him. At 6 feet 2 inches, Charlie had a tall body to fuel. He loved the idea of using his hand as a measuring guide. Not only was it convenient, but it was portion perfect. According to the palm of his hand, Charlie's poultry portion was closer to 6 ounces, not the usual 3–4 ounces. When I saw him one month later, he explained how much more satisfied he was with his portions. He'd dropped 18 pounds and had adjusted well to the idea of measuring his portions.

STAGE 2
Your Environment

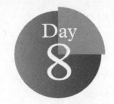

Right-Size Your Dishes

> Giant silverware makes the portions look smaller, so you don't feel guilty about eating so much!
>
> —Randy Glasbergen

Portion sizes aren't all that have gotten bigger over the years. Plates, bowls, glasses, mugs, and even utensils have too. Studies have consistently shown that people eat and drink more when using larger tableware.[1] To lose weight, you might want to do double duty with your tape measure and use it not only on your waist but on your plates as well.

Too much on your plate

The average dinner plate has grown in diameter since the 1950s, from 9 or 10 inches to 12 inches (and some are as large as 16 inches!). It may not sound like much of a difference, but for some people, having more room translates into permission to pile on the food. Researchers from the Cancer Council Western Australia discovered that a 12-inch plate holds about 54 percent more food than a 9.6-inch plate—even though the diameter of the plate increased by only 25 percent. And while it might not seem to make mathematical sense, a 9.6-inch plate holds about 630 calories' worth of food—570 *fewer* calories than a 12-inch plate, which holds an estimated 1,200 calories.[2]

There's a bit of psychology involved with plate size as well: The larger the plate, the smaller your portion looks, making it easy to misjudge and add too much food. Likewise, a small dish makes a portion look bigger. I recommend that you use a plate no larger than 10 inches or so for your meals. This one little trick can make a big difference.

If your dishes are large, you don't need to buy a new set. Just try some reverse psychology: Use your dinner plates for salad, a great way to boost your veggie consumption (and nutrient intake) and your smaller salad or dessert plates for your main course and side. Another option is to dust off Grandma's dishes for everyday use. Chances are they're portion perfect. When my client Susan, a fifty-four-year-old banker, started eating off her grandmother's plates, she ate less without even realizing it and lost weight. And watch those oversized bowls for pasta and cereal. Chances are the smaller bowl that comes with your set is a better choice.

Slice of Advice

If your food is overflowing from your plate, you've probably got—you guessed it—too much on your plate. Take some food off, and you'll have a healthier portion.

More than just appearances

Not only does smaller dishware give us the impression that we're eating more; it may also lead us to serve ourselves less. We often determine how much food to serve ourselves based on the size of our bowl or plate and even the serving spoon. And because so many of us are members of the clean-plate club, overserving can lead to overeating.

Plate size even dupes schoolchildren into eating more. Arcadia

University researchers gave first graders either a large, adult-sized plate or a small plate to use when serving themselves lunch. About 80 percent of the children with the large plate served themselves about 90 more calories (and ate about half of them) than those using the smaller plates.[3] The moral of the story: If you're having trouble losing weight, you may want to consider eating off smaller dishes.

Slice of Advice I know people who think it is fun to eat off of charger plates—those satellite dishes used under dinner plates to enhance a table setting. Chances are you're going to put too much on a charger plate and not realize it, and sabotaging your weight-loss goals is not fun. If you love eating off of large plates, use them for veggies.

Crystal clear

Wineglasses are another case in point. University of Cambridge researchers discovered that the volume of the average wineglass has swelled sevenfold since the 1700s—and most of that increase has taken place since the 1990s. This may be connected to the escalation in wine consumption in the United Kingdom in recent years, the researchers noted, but what is crystal clear is that people drink more wine when it's served in larger glasses.[4] The shape of the glass can also make a difference in how quickly you drink your alcoholic beverage. University of Bristol researchers found that people drank more quickly from a curved glass as opposed to a straight glass.[5]

Bite-Sized Goodie Stop signs and lights, it seems, are red for a reason. Swiss researchers found that the color red subconsciously acts as a stop signal even when it comes to food and drink. People ate less snack food and drank less from red plates and red-labeled cups when compared to people using blue or white tableware.[6]

To lose weight, you don't have to break out your childhood tea set. Just make small shifts at home and you won't even realize you're eating less. But do measure your plates (just once!) and opt for those smaller in circumference, unless you're filling up on freebies.

Wedge of Wisdom

My client Holly started using her china set, which had smaller plates and bowls than she was used to. After trying this for a week, her first comment to me was that she felt more satisfied with her portions. Eating off the nicer plates helped as well—she felt as if she were treating herself to an elegant meal.

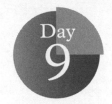

Declutter Your Kitchen

The remarkable thing about my mother is that for thirty years she served us nothing but leftovers. The original meal has never been found.

—Calvin Trillin

A messy and cluttered kitchen screams chaos, a chaotic environment makes us feel stressed, and stress may lead to overeating. The domino effect of countertops overcrowded with boxes of food, kitchen tables scattered with bills and paperwork, and kitchen drawers crammed with cooking utensils is weight gain. When your kitchen environment is disorderly, it interferes with your portion-control mind-set and may hurt your efforts to lose weight. Cluttered and chaotic environments may cause us to snack more, and there may even be a link between the mess, increased stress, and weight gain.[1] Even where and how we store our food affects what and how much we eat. Take a deep breath and relax. I've got some simple, no- or low-cost surefire ways to turn any kitchen into a haven of peace that inspires weight loss.

Is your kitchen stressing you out?

If your kitchen is stressing you out, it's time to get organized. Set aside a few hours to attack the project—or tackle it when the mood strikes you. Get the family to pitch in so it goes faster. Getting organized might mean tossing some stuff and buying a few new kitchen-organizing tools. Before bringing in anything new, I like to get rid of the old. Here are some suggestions:

Spices. Throw away old spices, combine duplicates, and consider whether you need a new spice rack.

Refrigerator and freezer. Toss expired and unhealthy items, combine duplicate condiments, and wash the shelves. Put single-serving treats in a bin toward the back. Keep fresh and frozen fruits and veggies front and center.

Countertops. Treat decluttering countertops as you would your workspace—take everything off and return only what's necessary. Store or give away infrequently used small appliances and cookbooks. Mount whatever you can on the wall. Most important, remove all food except for a bowl of your favorite fresh fruit. I'm a fan of apples and pears because they are simple—just wash and eat, no peeling necessary! Get in the habit of keeping the counter clean and clear.

Cupboards. Recycle chipped coffee mugs and glasses and arrange like items together. If time allows, change up the liners. Recycle storage containers that are missing lids. Stack containers neatly or replace with collapsible containers.

Drawers. Use drawer bins to organize knives, spatulas, and other items. Or set them in a large jar on the countertop. Perhaps treat yourself to a new set of kitchenware.

Pantry. Empty boxed and bagged foods into storage containers—clear for healthy items and opaque for treats. Walking into a pantry full of packages is an assault to the senses. Containers help you see what items you're running low on and give your pantry a clean, fresh feel. Place portion-perfect scoops into containers of nuts and other treats. Use oversized jars to store single-serve packs or baggies of snacks such as nuts.

Catchall space. Put mail, purse, change, keys, and other miscellaneous stuff in a designated spot so it doesn't land on the kitchen table or countertop—and so it's always in the same spot when you need it.

Portion-control station. Place commonly used items within reach—especially those you use to control your portions. This might include food scale, measuring cups, measuring spoons, and portion-ready bowls and containers, as well as different-sized baggies you can use to divvy up large packages of food. We'll talk more about this in Day #10: Cook Like a Portion Pro (page 111).

Simple kitchen organizers

You don't need to have a kitchen the size of the Taj Mahal to properly store everything. Some of the tools available for organizing small spaces are ingenious:

- Sliding shelf organizers
- Drawer organizers
- Baskets and bins
- Cart with wheels
- Pots-and-pans hanger
- Retractable cookbook stand
- Wire racks or tension rods for cutting boards and baking sheets

Bite-Sized Goodie In addition to clutter, chaos can come in the form of people and noise (aka family). If mealtimes are louder and crazier than you'd like, take yourself to your happy place. Recall a memory of a good time or put on some soft music to change the mood.

Make some moves

Once your kitchen is clean and orderly, strive to keep it tidy. Stay mindful of what goes on your countertop and how you store your food. Vow to bring in only healthy foods. And make some moves or adjustments. Tweaking things here and there in your kitchen can make "pounds" of difference.

Keep healthy foods such as fresh fruit on your kitchen counter. When you walk into the kitchen looking for a snack, you're more likely to grab what's easily accessible, so showcase something healthy. Fruits are on the freebies list, so keep them visible. A bowl of fresh fruit not only looks appetizing but also brightens up a room.

Put the cereal and chips away, even the whole-grain varieties. Put the cereal in the cupboard where you can't see it. Whole-grain cereal is good for you, but you know the mantra—eat too much and you'll gain weight. Same rule applies to popcorn and chips, even the healthy versions!

Conceal the candy. Place candy, cookies, and other treats in opaque containers. Take it a step further and make them hard to reach, either on top shelves or in the deep recesses of your cupboard. Out of sight, out of mind.

Follow the rule of one. Keep only one bag of candy and one type of cookie in your kitchen at a time. The more variety we have, the more we tend to eat. This concept works great with fruits and vegetables. But when it comes to candy and junk food, one selection is more than enough.[2]

Stock your fridge with fresh vegetables for snacks. Keep a regular supply of baby carrots, celery, or red peppers in your fridge in eyesight. Experiment with new veggies too—jicama, for example, makes for a crunchy munchie. When you have time, wash and chop or cut your veggies and place them in clear bowls. Or chop extra

WELLNESS KITCHENS

If you plan on redesigning your kitchen anytime soon, consider the Wellness Kitchen. A recent trend in kitchen design merges environment, health, and lifestyle to accommodate today's cooks, many of whom prefer fresh produce over processed foods. Whereas post–World War II kitchens included plenty of cupboards for processed foods and were walled off from other rooms, Wellness Kitchens focus on open shelving, room to grow fresh produce, plenty of ventilation, an outdoor cooking space, and an open floor plan to facilitate socializing.[3]

when you cook a meal. When you're hungry or in a rush, you've got healthy choices at your fingertips.

Put a date on your leftovers. To avoid forgetting how old your leftovers are, use a dry-erase marker on your baggies or clear containers to date your leftover meals and snacks. Don't leave it up to your memory to remember.

Have any mirrors in your dining area? Don't look at them when you eat. Researchers at Nagoya University in Japan found that we eat more food when looking in a mirror, just as we do when we dine with others.[4] Turns out even our reflection is good company!

Clean countertops and organized spaces clear the way for weight loss. If you don't believe me, give it a try. You've nothing to lose except weight.

Wedge of Wisdom

My client Leslie, like many city dwellers, has a small kitchen. She has two school-age boys who like a snack when they get home from school. Short of pantry space, and to make it easy for the kids, Leslie kept junk food sitting out on the counter but nibbled on it herself. I suggested she get different types of containers—opaque for unhealthy and clear for healthy—and that she keep only fruit on the counter. These two little tricks made a world of difference. She nibbled far less, and her kids ate fruit when they got home!

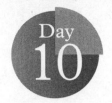

Cook Like a Portion Pro

The biggest seller is cookbooks and the second is diet books—how not to eat what you've just learned how to cook.

—Andy Rooney

Americans are relying more and more on food prepared outside the home, a pattern that has been linked to obesity.[1] When you eat home-cooked meals, you eat less, eat healthier, save money, and are more likely to stick to your food plan.[2] At home, measuring portions is also superconvenient—especially when you have the right tools. And you tend to get better at estimating portion sizes for when you do eat out.

Measuring portion sizes at home once in a while is key to weight loss. Large portion sizes may have started in restaurants, but they have infiltrated the home. We've become accustomed to seeing oversize portions when eating out, and now, no matter where we eat, big portions may feel like the new normal.

I advocate for cooking at home as often as possible, or at least a few meals each week. But portion control should be fun. So here I show you some unique portion-control gadgets that make measuring fun and easy. I also offer some great portion-friendly cooking tips that can turn meal prep into a labor of love, if it isn't already.

Portion props to the rescue

Companies have been coming out with all sorts of portion-savvy products to support people trying to lose weight through portion control. And researchers are finding that this type of support works. In a study at Spain's University of Navarra, obese people given guided crockery sets (plates divided into sections as a way to measure portions) and calibrated serving spoons (measuring spoons used for serving) found them easy to use and "potentially effective" for weight loss, especially when it came to controlling starch servings, including chips and potatoes. When using these tools, participants also ate more nonstarchy vegetables.[3]

Measuring cups and spoons. These are your can't-live-without staples. Buy stackable stainless steel or plastic measuring cups and spoons for easy storage. You can even get collapsible ones that take up hardly any space. Have multiple sets on hand so you can separate them and leave them in your containers of rice, oatmeal, popcorn, and dried legumes for quick and accurate measuring. I suggest a set for measuring liquids as well as a set for measuring solid ingredients. Liquids easily overflow from measuring cups made for solids.

Kitchen scales. A food scale is convenient for weighing fish, chicken, lean meats and other foods by the ounce. Some digital versions even calculate nutrition information (although I'm somewhat suspicious of the accuracy of such information).

Plates, bowls, cups, glasses, and mugs. Product designers have stepped up to the plate when it comes to portion-control dishware, with everything from plates etched with designs to mark off portions to bowls rimmed on the inside with lines indicating serving size—like a built-in measuring cup. You can even buy wineglasses marked with fill lines. Portion-control dishware is a good reminder to pay attention to your portions.

Spray bottles. Fill these reusable dispensers with extra-virgin olive oil to spray on your salads, veggies, and frying pans. These top prepackaged cooking sprays because they're missing added chemicals, and you still minimize how much fat you add to a meal, which helps you to stay within your fat budget.

Food containers. Use these to store portion-perfect meals you cook ahead of time and freeze. They're also great for storing fruits, vegetables, snacks, homemade salad dressings, and more. To remind you how much each container holds, label them accordingly. You can purchase many different-sized containers ranging from ¼ cup up to 7 cups. I use both glass and plastic containers. I store the glass in the fridge and travel with the plastic. If you use containers coded by food group—by the color of either the container or the lid—you can quickly find what you need from each food group. For instance, use 1-cup containers for starch; ½-cup containers for meats; and ¼-cup containers for fats; and put nonstarchy veggies and fruits in the biggest containers. When you're ready to eat, just empty the appropriate containers onto your plate for a portion-perfect meal.

Ingenious inventions. Blenders, juicers, spiralizers, and air popcorn poppers will make your life easier if you like to make smoothies, fresh vegetable juice, homemade zoodles, and your own oil-free popcorn (instead of buying the more processed microwave popcorn).

Water bottles. If carrying around a gallon jug or large mason jar is not your style, look for water bottles with measuring lines, filters, or even a place to infuse your favorite fruit flavor into your H_2O. Toting a water bottle with you wherever you go encourages you to stay hydrated and get in your 64 ounces a day.

See Appendix D (page 289) for a list of more fun portion props, along with my top picks.

Unless you're sharing a whole avocado with others, you're bound to have leftovers. To keep your leftover avocado from turning brown, squeeze an acidic agent such as lemon or lime juice on the exposed face of the avocado. You can do the same for mashed or sliced avocado and even guacamole. Cover with plastic wrap or store in an airtight container in the refrigerator for up to a day.

Make it healthy *and* portion ready

When you cook at home, you know what goes into your food and how much goes on your plate. Cooking at home *with confidence* makes you less likely to consume the ultraprocessed foods we talk about in Day #12: Think "Whole-istically" (page 122).[4] But not everyone has the time or inclination to cook. Whether you're a gourmet foodie or you can't stand the heat, here are some foolproof portion-control cooking tips to boost your confidence in the kitchen and your weight loss as well.

Make it muffin-sized. The standard muffin pan is the perfect instrument for pulling off a host of recipes that go beyond batter—and all made to fit. I'm talking portion-perfect veggie omelets, oatmeal cups, yogurt parfaits, your favorite potato dish, and much, much more, single-serve style. Just Google "muffin pan recipes" and take your pick of healthy concoctions. You'll have portion-ready food on hand for several days.

Stuff it. Who says stuffed peppers have to be green and full of beef? For nutritional variety, use red or yellow peppers. But don't stop there. Replace half the lean ground beef with chopped mushrooms, celery, carrots, spinach, and onion—or whatever you have on hand. Or make it vegetarian by stuffing your peppers with a homemade stew of veggies and legumes. Use brown and wild rice instead of white and you've got an entire healthy meal at the ready.

Cook it in a cup. A coffee mug and a microwave can give you an (almost) instant, portion-ready meal at home or the office—everything from omelets to burrito bowls, bean dishes, quinoa, and meat loaf—often without added fat, salt, or sugar. Google "coffee mug recipes" for hundreds of clever ideas—even single-serving desserts.

Try something new. If you're in a cooking rut, browse through recipe books, look online for a new take on an old dish, or venture into your local farmers' market with the intention of buying a fruit or vegetable you've never cooked before.

Make your own salad dressing. To keep your salad pure and healthy, make your own dressing with extra-virgin olive oil. Add a splash of lemon, your favorite herbs and spices, fresh garlic, mustard, and balsamic or apple cider vinegar for some instant zest. Play around with the exact proportions that taste best to you. Bear in mind that vinegar, mustard, and lemon cut the calories in your dressing considerably. If you want bigger portions, consider adding more of these ingredients.

Cooking at home makes it easier for you to stay on the Plan, but it shouldn't feel like a life sentence. Make it fun by creating a portion-friendly kitchen, with portion props at the ready. An added bonus: The more you cook at home, the more dining out feels like a real treat.

Wedge of Wisdom

Carole, a thirty-year-old single graduate student, was never much of a cook and tended to order in a lot. In her mind, cooking was a superelaborate affair she would tackle only when she had company. To help her cut back on the amount of restaurant food she was eating, we discussed how to prepare a few simple meals at home. She got herself some portion props and fun gadgets and started making grilled chicken and fish, spiraled vegetable dishes, and some healthy grains such as soba noodles and quinoa. While she continued ordering takeout on occasion, she reported enjoying her home-cooked meals more.

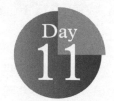

Prepare the Perfect Plate

There is a difference between eating and drinking for
strength and from mere gluttony.

—Henry David Thoreau

The perfect plate showcases the different food groups in proper
proportions. The simplest of all plate arrangements is the divide-
and-conquer approach: Fill half your plate with colorful nonstarchy
veggies and fruit; one-quarter with a healthy protein such as fish,
poultry, legumes, eggs, or lean beef; and the remaining quarter with
a smart starch such as brown rice, quinoa, or sweet potato. Dividing
your meal up by food groups is a useful way to control your portion sizes. It also means you won't be staring at an empty plate. The
perfect plate is always a full plate.

Not everything you eat, however, comfortably falls into one food
group. Stews, stir-fries, chilies, pasta dishes, stuffed peppers, and
even peanut butter sandwiches are mixed dishes, or a blend of food
groups. Chicken soup, for example, might include noodles (starch),
carrots and celery (veggies), and chicken (poultry). To estimate how
much you're eating from each food group, visually take your meal
apart. For example:

Peanut butter sandwich =
2 slices of whole-grain bread (2 servings of starch) +
1 tablespoon peanut butter (1 serving of fats)

Homemade veggie pizza =
1 large whole-grain tortilla (2 servings of starch) + ⅓ cup
shredded cheese (1 serving of dairy) + broccoli, spinach, red
peppers, and onion (nonstarchy vegetables) + ½ cup tomato
sauce (nonstarchy vegetable)

Vegetarian black bean chili and sweet potato =
½ cup beans (1 serving of meat alternative) + ½ can diced
tomatoes (2 servings of nonstarchy vegetables) + 1 sweet
potato (2 servings of starches) + 1 tablespoon olive oil
(1 serving of fats) + onion, garlic, spices, lime juice

FINALLY FULL, FINALLY SLIM
PORTION PLATE

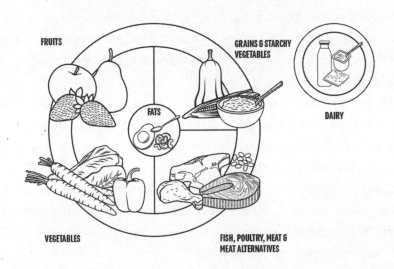

Preparing the perfect plate is not meant to be rocket science. If your piece of chicken is 4–5 ounces instead of 3, don't sweat it. If your portion is closer to 10 ounces, on the other hand, scale back and replace the extra space on your plate with more veggies. Dividing your meal up by food groups is brilliant. You see when a portion is out of whack and can quickly correct it. This works provided that the size of your plate is not skewing the math. We talked about plate size at great length in Day #8: Right-Size Your Dishes (page 101): If your plates, bowls, and mugs are extra-large, use the dinner plate for your salad and the salad plate for the rest of your meal.

To save calories, prepare your plate *before* you sit down to eat. We tend to eat more when food is served family style, or on the table and within reach. When the food is in front of us, it's almost too easy to go for second helpings.

A balancing act

When it comes to getting the right balance of macronutrients (protein, fats, and carbohydrates), I have a few pointers.

Fats. Eating a small portion of fat with a meal helps you stay full throughout the day. Choose healthy fats and avoid doubling up. Eating more than one added fat at a meal is how a lot of my clients get into trouble. For instance, enjoy an avocado or nuts in your salad, but not both—maybe put the avocado in your salad and save the nuts for a snack. Fats have more than double the calories of protein or carbohydrates, so amounts do count. Remember your portions, even for healthy fats.

Carbohydrates. If you have a hard time portioning starch, include it in one or two meals, not all three. If you have oatmeal at breakfast, opt for a salad at lunch instead of a sandwich. You can still have a sweet potato or a cup of quinoa, farro, or wild rice with dinner.

Protein. Protein helps with weight loss in several ways. It signals the brain that you are full. It also helps to stabilize blood sugar, which may help to curb sugar cravings, so eat it throughout the day in thoughtful portion sizes. I recommend eating a protein-rich food at each meal and as part of an afternoon snack. High-protein foods include fish, poultry, meat, legumes, and some dairy. Vegetables, whole grains, nuts, and seeds also provide some protein. For instance, you could include an egg or yogurt for breakfast, a salad with legumes for lunch, some cottage cheese, nuts, or hummus as part of an afternoon snack, and chicken or fish for dinner.

If you eat too much protein, like with carbs or fats, you will gain weight. Excess calories are excess calories. They don't just disappear. So stick to healthy portions. It's very easy to eat at least 6–8 ounces of protein when you go out for dinner. On days you plan to eat fish, chicken, or lean meat at a restaurant, choose plant-based proteins earlier in the day.

Get extra mileage out of your portions

While you focus on losing weight, you can improve your memory and gut health, too. When selecting what to put on your plate, keep the following foods in mind.

Food for thought. Salmon, avocados, blueberries, dark leafy greens, walnuts, black and green tea, turmeric, yogurt, beets, and eggs are known to power brain cells and improve memory. Many people avoid eating the yolk of an egg because it's high in cholesterol, but the yellow center holds most of the fat, B vitamins, and choline—which are good for the brain.

Fermented food. For thousands of years, people have used yeast or bacteria to ferment food—everything from beans, fruits, and dairy to grains, vegetables, and meats. Fermentation preserves food and changes up the flavor and texture. An added benefit is that the microbes in fermented foods boost gut health, reduce inflammation, and may even help with weight loss. Enjoy yogurt, kefir, kombucha, sauerkraut, tempeh, kimchi, or miso either with a meal or as a snack. Even sourdough bread is fermented, and many people who are gluten intolerant are able to tolerate sourdough bread, much to their surprise.

Bite-Sized Goodie Enjoy a souped-up appetizer. Vegetable-based soups are a great way to start a meal. They're filling and nutritious, and according to Penn State researchers, eating soup before a meal helped to reduce calorie intake by 20 percent![1]

Slice of Advice Double the size of your oatmeal by adding lots of fruit. I love adding a chopped apple and blueberries to uncooked oatmeal before cooking it up. You get an oversized bowl of yummy oatmeal with warm fruit. And how sweet it is.

To prepare the perfect plate, be cognizant of the different food groups and know your portions. Preparing the perfect plate gets easier with practice. Before long, you won't even need to think about it.

Wedge of Wisdom

Daniella, one of my blog readers, shared with me that a friend of hers (whom we'll call Janice) lost more than 50 pounds just by following my advice to prepare a colorful plate. For years, Janice had equated weight loss with small serving sizes. She felt deprived. When she began preparing a full, colorful plate of food, she began to equate weight loss with abundance. She looked forward to facing a plate full of cheerful, colorful vegetables at every meal. Suddenly, dieting became enjoyable. For the first time in more than a decade, Janice's weight fell below the 200-pound mark.

Think "Whole-istically"

We are living in a world today where lemonade is made
from artificial flavors and furniture polish is made from real
lemons.

—Alfred E. Neuman

The Plan is about more than losing weight. It's also about improving health. That means choosing nutritious whole and minimally processed foods with as few unhealthy additives as possible, as often as you can. Eating mostly whole and minimally processed food has been proven to give you the best chance at weight loss, good health, and even a longer life. Ultraprocessed foods, on the other hand, promote overconsumption. Tasty (because added sodium, fat, refined starches, and sugars make them hyperpalatable), overly processed foods can lead to excess pounds and extra visits to the doctor. The evidence is overwhelming.[1]

Most of the chronic diseases prevalent today were not nearly as common before processed foods began replacing homemade everything in the early 1900s. Generations of Americans have grown up on processed foods, and our health records show it: Obesity, high blood pressure, type 2 diabetes, and gut issues, including colon cancer, are more prevalent than ever, all in the name of progress.[2]

Americans aren't the only ones suffering. Researchers from the University of São Paulo in Brazil who looked at the prevalence of obesity in nineteen European countries found a strong link between obesity and households that regularly bought ultraprocessed foods such as soft drinks, mass-produced packaged breads, and chicken nuggets.[3]

In an attempt to fight chronic health conditions, a return to eating real food in its purest, whole form makes good sense.

The spectrum

Whole food is basically intact, in its natural, whole form. No one has canned or boxed it or added salt, sugar, fat, or chemicals to enhance color, flavor, or shelf life.[4] Whole foods include vegetables, fruits, nuts, legumes, eggs, meat, fish, and poultry—almost everything on the Plan.

Minimally processed foods do not contain large amounts of added fat, salt, or sugar. Examples of minimally processed foods are oil, spices (without additives), and stewed tomatoes. Bagged or chopped veggies; frozen fruit and vegetables; and store-bought guacamole, hummus, and tahini are also good examples. They've been prepped for your convenience, but they don't display a lengthy list of additives, most of which you can't pronounce. Minimally processed foods retain most of their nutritional properties, and many are as nutritious as they are in their unprocessed form.[5] It's more than fine to eat minimally processed foods. And as best-selling author Michael Pollan writes in his book *Food Rules*, "Don't eat anything your great-grandmother wouldn't recognize as food."[6]

If a label contains several ingredients you can't pronounce, leave it on the shelf. You're better off looking for a less-processed item or making it yourself.

SAY GOOD-BYE TO ARTIFICIAL TRANS FATS

In 2018, the FDA began clamping down on food manufacturers to eliminate artificial trans fats from their products, found mostly in unhealthy foods such as baked goods, fried foods, refrigerator dough, frozen pizza crusts, nondairy coffee creamer, and stick margarines. Artificial trans fats are created by adding hydrogen to vegetable oil in the manufacturing process. Manufacturers use them for commercially processed baked goods because they don't spoil as quickly as other fats and have a longer shelf life. According to the FDA, removing artificial trans fats from the food supply will prevent thousands of heart attacks and deaths every year. But be careful— some food manufacturers are replacing trans fats with tropical oils high in saturated fat, which is also known to raise total cholesterol.[7]

Moving beyond minimally processed foods, we begin to inch our way toward the far end of the spectrum—ultraprocessed foods. Examples of processed and heavily processed items include store-bought cookies and cakes, lunch meats and sausages, soy burgers, veggie sausages, and frozen dinners. These products contain added sugar, salt, and fat, as well as preservatives and other artificial ingredients. While the food industry sells a lot of ultraprocessed foods, it is trending toward offering healthier, less-processed ready-to-eat foods, such as quinoa and bean dishes and other whole-grain meals that are low in sodium and contain few added ingredients. This is good news.

Most of us are going to buy processed foods some of the time as a matter of convenience. When you do, read the labels and buy the healthiest options. Choose the tomato sauce lowest in sodium and added sugar (yes, some tomato sauces have added sugar) or frozen carrots without sauce instead of frozen carrots in a sauce, for instance. Selecting minimally processed foods takes minimal effort once you get the hang of it.

While I suggest you cut back on highly processed foods, if you do eat them on occasion, here are some quick tricks to boost nutrition and increase satisfaction:

- Add frozen, whole, or precut veggies; legumes (lentils, chickpeas, black beans); or nuts (peanuts, cashews, almonds, walnuts, pecans, pistachios, pine nuts) to a frozen entrée.
- Top a frozen pizza with spinach and broccoli.
- Mix pureed beans or hummus into a jar of marinara sauce.
- Add veggies and chickpeas to your frozen pasta dinner.

Shake the sodium habit

Most Americans get too much sodium in their diet, but most of it is not coming from saltshakers. "Salt" is the common term for sodium chloride, which is made of 40 percent sodium and 60 percent chloride. Sodium also acts as a preservative, thickener, and flavor enhancer, so most ultraprocessed foods and some restaurant meals are high in sodium. Most Americans consume about 3,400 milligrams of sodium daily.[8] The *Dietary Guidelines* recommend limiting sodium intake to no more than 2,300 milligrams each day, or about 1 teaspoon of salt. That'd be easy to do if we saw all the salt we consume. But our saltshaker is not typically the culprit. The top sources of sodium in our diet are breads, cold cuts, pizza, burritos, tacos, sandwiches, savory snacks, and cheese.[9]

Most of us consume sodium without even knowing it. But excessive salt intake comes with a price when it comes to the heart because it can cause water retention and lead to high blood pressure.[10] To cut back on sodium intake, read the ingredients list on food labels and compare the sodium content of different brands to make smarter choices.

Here are some tips and tricks to reduce your sodium intake:

- If you eat out often or buy a lot of processed food, don't add salt when cooking at home.
- Use flavor enhancers such as spices and herbs, onions, garlic, and scallions.
- Choose products labeled "low sodium."
- Always read the label for sodium levels.

Bite-Sized Goodie Packaging that shouts "Eat me!" is likely just working really hard to get your attention and distract you from considering the product's nutritional value, as my New York University colleague Marion Nestle writes in her award-winning book *Food Politics*. Fun, attractive, or loud packaging, along with many health claims, is all about the sell, which is quite possibly a disguise for poor nutrition.[11]

Herbs and seasonings add flavor to food, but did you know they can lower blood pressure and promote heart health? Researchers from the Army Medical University in China discovered that subjects who preferred spices consumed less salt and had lower blood pressure than people who shied away from flavoring their foods with anything other than salt.[12]

Love Your Heart

Seasoning your favorite foods with spices not only enhances flavor but boosts your nutrient intake and can help fight the aging process. Turmeric and ginger, for example, contain anti-inflammatory properties, while cumin contains antibacterial properties. As an added benefit, seasoning your foods with spices helps to reduce your need to use added sugar and salt.

Replace highly processed dressings and marinades you buy in the store with a homemade sauce of olive oil, vinegar, fresh lemon, herbs, and garlic.

When to buy organic

Some fruits and vegetables soak up more pesticides than others during cultivation. To reduce your exposure to pesticides, you may want to consider buying organic produce when possible. The nonprofit Environmental Working Group (EWG) creates two lists annually to help you determine when buying organic may make the best sense: the Dirty Dozen and the Clean Fifteen.

The Dirty Dozen lists the fruits and veggies with the most chemical residue *after* being washed or peeled. Strawberries, spinach, nectarines, apples, grapes, peaches, cherries, pears, tomatoes, celery, potatoes, and sweet bell peppers top the list. Strive to buy organic when purchasing these produce varieties. If, for whatever reason, you are not able to buy organic produce, you are still far better off eating conventionally grown produce than not eating produce at all.

The Clean Fifteen lists the fruits and veggies with the least amount of pesticide residue. Don't feel pressured to buy organic avocados, sweet corn, pineapples, cabbage, onions, sweet peas, papayas, asparagus, mangos, eggplant, honeydew melon, kiwifruit, cantaloupe, cauliflower, and grapefruit. Visit ewg.org to view the most recent lists.[13]

You can take this a step further and buy locally grown produce. It's fresher (because it doesn't have to travel halfway across the country in a truck) and supports your community.

More important than anything, to reduce your exposure to pesticides, whether you opt for organic or conventionally grown produce, it's important to wash your fruits and vegetables under warm running water and discard any outer leaves before eating and cooking.

Add a healthy decade to your life

Consistently eating whole or minimally processed foods helps us live longer. Ohio University researchers found that people were less likely to die early if they regularly consumed a diet consisting primarily of whole grains, vegetables, fruits, nuts, and fish over a twelve-year period. Even small dietary changes made a big difference:

- Cut out 1 serving of red or processed meat a day and go meat-less by replacing it with lentils, chickpeas, or black beans.
- Eat a palm full of raw nuts for a dose of heart-healthy fats.
- Eat some protein (yogurt, eggs, nut butter) at breakfast and you may end up saving calories later in the day.
- Eat at home instead of a restaurant or fast-food joint at least once a week and save calories, saturated fat, and sodium.

People who made these changes were able to stick with them. The best news? It's never too late to start.[14]

The old adage "You are what you eat" still holds true today. Any diet that promotes weight loss should also promote health. The more you turn to whole foods, the better and more satisfied you'll feel. Before you know it, the thought of eating a heavily processed Danish or frozen pizza won't appeal. Now, that's what I call progress.

Wedge of Wisdom

Jane, a busy full-time lawyer, followed a diet composed mostly of frozen entrées, canned soups, and processed meats. She felt that she didn't have time to cook and prepare healthy foods. She rarely felt satisfied unless she ate two frozen entrées for dinner and junk for dessert. I suggested she eliminate some of the highly processed foods and helped her boost the nutrition levels of the processed foods she was eating. She stocked up on frozen veggies and fruits, canned beans, bags of salad greens, cherry tomatoes, baby carrots, and other foods requiring minimal preparation. She started adding frozen veggies and a salad to her entrées. And instead of eating cookies after dinner, she nuked frozen berries in the microwave and had a satisfying snack. She was shocked to see how easy it was to add healthful foods to her diet, and she lost 20 pounds in the process!

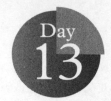

Fill Up on Freebies

Vegetables are a must on a diet. I suggest carrot cake, zucchini bread, and pumpkin pie.

—Jim Davis

When people try to lose weight, they are usually told that they have to eliminate certain foods and eat less. They start out feeling deprived before they even have their first meal. Dieting becomes something they must endure rather than something to anticipate. I want you to look forward to your meals, to losing weight, and to feeling healthy. That's why nonstarchy vegetables and fruit are freebies in the Plan. Fruits and veggies don't have many calories (so there's no need to meticulously count them), they're filling and nutritious, and most people don't get enough of them.

Take advantage of freebies, and you won't miss what you used to have on your plate before you started the Plan. Penn State professor Dr. Barbara Rolls and colleagues found that we get used to eating a certain *volume* of food as opposed to a certain number of calories. We tend to care more about *how much* is on our plate than we do about *what's* on it.[1] In other words, you'll likely feel just as satisfied eating a plate full of veggies as you would if you ate a steak that covered your entire plate.

It's a concept known as crowding out: Eat generous portions of nonstarchy veggies and fruit and you will no longer want a cookie or ice cream cone. You won't need a ginormous bowl of pasta if you add lots of colorful vegetables and fresh tomato sauce.

Here's another reason to eat your veggies. Eating produce regularly may even improve mood, motivation, and vitality. And it doesn't take long to feel these changes. Researchers from the University of Otago in New Zealand who gave young adults fruits and veggies to eat daily for two weeks showed improved vitality, were more motivated, and felt more curious and creative.[2]

Veg out with veggies

Here are a few ways to put more veggies in your life.

Eat freebies first. Eating a salad before your meal reduces your calorie intake. You're also likely to increase the amount of veggies you eat with your entrée by almost 25 percent.[3] You can also add veggies to your soup or put crudités (vegetables and dip) out before a meal.

Choose foods you enjoy. Rather than try to force-feed yourself a veggie you don't like, choose one that you do enjoy. And instead of concentrating on foods you should avoid, focus on foods you can eat.[4]

Serve them separate. Put your veggies on a separate plate entirely, if need be, so they don't compete with more enticing foods. Researchers learned that when all you see on your plate is veggies, you eat more of them.[5]

Keep cool. Fill your freezer with freebies. They will last for a couple of months, so you will have them on hand if you run out of fresh varieties. University of California–Davis researchers found that, overall, frozen fruits and vegetables are packed with just as many nutrients as their fresh counterparts.[6] I always keep my freezer stocked with frozen fruits and veggies even though I buy fresh produce regularly.

Dress down. You already know that foods in the fats group, as well as those in treats and sweets, are not freebies. So don't disqualify a freebie by adding too much dressing, sauce, or sugar. Enjoy your fruit unsweetened—frozen grapes taste great, as do baked apples sprinkled with cinnamon and nutmeg. Use a little olive or sesame oil or your favorite homemade marinade on steamed broccoli. A small amount goes a long way—and you may find you prefer tasting the actual fruit or vegetable as nature intended.

 Limit your reliance on frozen meals because some are crazy high in sodium. But consider using healthier and lower-sodium versions to adjust to realistic portion sizes. Take advantage of the home-delivery meals that may be available where you live. A study published in *Obesity* showed that, when combined with behavioral counseling, ready meals (packaged, frozen, or delivered fresh to your home) can help you lose weight because they are portion appropriate.[7] Add veggies of your own to increase the fullness factor.

Mix it up

Freebies aren't just for salads. You can add them into other food groups. If you aren't a fan of fruits and vegetables, disguise the taste by pureeing them and adding them to soups, sauces, and casseroles. Penn State researchers found that adults who incorporated pureed veggies into their meals significantly reduced their calorie intake while increasing their vegetable consumption.[8] Freebies easily add volume to other foods and can even replace pasta, rice, and more. Following are some ideas:

- Replace half your ground beef with chopped mushrooms.
- Try rice made from cauliflower. It looks (and tastes) like white rice, but it's just veggies, so you can eat a larger portion than you could if eating real rice. If you buy prepackaged cauliflower rice, read the label to ensure you're not getting any hidden salt, sugar, added fat, or other sneaky sources of calories.
- Bulk up a quarter plate of whole-wheat pasta with sauce and veggies. Cut up broccoli, onions, mushrooms, bell peppers, carrots, or whatever you have on hand.
- Replace pasta with spiraled zucchini, sweet potato, or beets. Use a spiralizer or buy spiraled veggies already prepped in the prepared salad or freezer section of your grocery store. Top with olive oil or fresh tomato sauce and grated cheese, and you've got it made.
- Add shredded produce to your vegetable repertoire. In addition to shredded cabbage, broccoli and Brussels sprouts slaw taste yummy. Enjoy them cooked and drizzled with toasted sesame oil.
- Add pureed veggies to soups, sauces, and casseroles.
- Replace hamburger buns, sandwich bread, or wraps with lettuce or spinach.
- Add apples, bananas, strawberries, or blueberries, along with a tablespoon of walnuts or almonds, to your bowl of oatmeal, ready-to-eat cereal, or yogurt to make a supersized portion without a lot of calories.
- Add spinach, kale, tomatoes, mushrooms, onions, or any other veggie to your omelet or frittata, or cook them as a side for poached or fried eggs.
- Add greens, cucumbers, and tomatoes to your wrap or sandwich.
- Bulk up stews, soups, and casseroles with chopped nonstarchy veggies.
- Blend up a green vegetable drink with your favorite veggies.

- Make a frozen drink for dessert. I love the combination of ½ pear, ½ cup blueberries, and 1 cup fat-free milk or unsweetened vanilla almond milk, plus 1 tablespoon peanut powder for flavor. Add lots of ice for bulk. It's healthier than ice cream.

 Adding vegetables to an unhealthy meal doesn't make it healthy. Dr. Alexander Chernev from Northwestern University found that people perceived a burger with three celery sticks to be lower in calories than the burger alone.[9] I like to call this wishful thinking.

As you get into the mind-set of filling up on freebies, you'll begin to notice new and fun opportunities to incorporate them into your life. Be creative! Make your freebies exciting. When you fill your life with abundance, there's no room for feelings of deprivation.

Wedge of Wisdom

Julie entertains clients a lot, which means she eats out a lot. When others in her party order dessert, Julie feels obligated to join them. To maintain the weight she's worked so hard to reach, she orders one biscotto and a colorful bowl of berries and leaves the restaurant feeling light and satisfied. In the summer, she takes advantage of fresh melon in season. This is a perfect example of pumping up the volume with freebies.

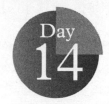

Shop Like a Chef

I accidentally went grocery shopping on an empty stomach
and now I'm the proud owner of aisle 7.

—Author unknown

Remember this statement: *Whatever you bring into your kitchen,
you will eat.* You may not think it applies to you, but it applies to
everyone. Weight loss begins at the grocery store. For this reason, I
encourage you to shop like a chef.

Chefs take food and grocery shopping seriously. They compare
and look for quality. They don't settle, at least not on a regular basis.
They carefully select ingredients that will pack a punch. Ripe, juicy
fruits, fresh vegetables, and whole grains top their shopping list,
along with legumes, fish, poultry, lean meat, nuts, dairy, and spices.
Chefs go for nutrition, color, balance, taste, and quality. And they
always consider how many people they'll be serving—and are therefore mindful about *portion size.*

Six essential ingredients

Before you head to the supermarket, put on your chef's hat and consider these six essential "ingredients" for shopping like a chef:

Portion size. Buy single servings of high-calorie foods such as nuts and treats and sweets, since you'll likely stop eating when your unit is gone.[1] Because buying in bulk can be cheaper and more environmentally friendly than buying in single servings, an alternative is to divide and conquer. Break down bulk items into single servings using baggies or small containers you can grab as you go. Separate and freeze large packages of fish, poultry, and meat by portion size.

Nutrition. Look for foods that give you more bang for your buck in terms of nutrients: fresh or frozen fruits and veggies, salmon (omega-3s), legumes (plant protein and fiber), and, as always, whole instead of refined grains.

Color. Buy fruits and veggies from all the colors of the rainbow (including white!) to ensure you're getting a variety of nutrients. Look for deep, rich hues that will turn a plate of food into an incredibly satisfying meal—as well as a piece of art.

Balance. Include all six food groups. Because fruits and veggies should fill half your plate, they should be half of your groceries too. Be sure to also include protein-rich foods such as fish, chicken, beans, legumes, eggs, and dairy products as well as whole grains and healthy fats.

Taste. Herbs and spices can go a long way toward making food taste better, and when you like what you're eating, you feel more satisfied. Some spices have added health benefits. Look for flavorful spices with no additives. Don't be afraid to experiment.

Quality. Quality goes hand in hand with nutrition, and choosing quality over quantity is one way to address oversized portions. Quality foods are fresh, have little or no additives and preservatives, and are not overflowing with fat, sugar, or salt. They fill you up with nutrients, not empty calories, so you are satisfied with a normal portion that doesn't leave you hankering for more. So look for whole or minimally processed foods.

Bite-Sized Goodie Every day, Americans toss 30–40 percent of their food because they overbuy at the grocery store or put too much on their plate. Planning at least a few meals, knowing what an adequate portion size looks like, and shopping with a list help you better gauge how much food you will likely consume between regular trips to the grocery store. A win-win for waist and waste.[2]

Don't leave home without it

Preparation is the hallmark of a savvy shopper, and, coupons aside, a shopper's single most important preparation tool is the list. A shopping list ensures that your kitchen is regularly stocked with healthy foods you can pick and choose from to create your next balanced meal. Lists keep you focused on what you need and rein you in during a weak moment in the cookie aisle.

Keep a running shopping list of items you need for a meal plan, new recipe, go-to snacks, and nearly depleted staples. I like to write items down on a small notepad, and before heading to the store I snap a picture of it in case I can't find it when I'm in the store. Use whatever method works best for you—a magnetic notepad you keep on the fridge, a notes folder on your smartphone (which you'll likely have with you), or your favorite app. If you order groceries online, take advantage of the store's built-in running shopping list.

From now on, you'll be shopping with intention and a plan, whenever possible. And it's not always going to be possible. But you have a plan for that, too. It's called your pantry.

Stock up and chill out

Nothing makes cooking and grocery shopping easier than having a kitchen well stocked with staples. When you run low on something, simply add the item to your shopping list and you haven't missed a beat. On those days when you're too busy to shop, you can turn to your staples and avert an unplanned restaurant meal or a drive through the fast-food lane.

Must-have pantry items

Healthy starches: Sweet potatoes, winter squash, and potatoes; kasha; quinoa; farro; soba noodles; brown and wild rice; whole-grain cereals, bread, tortillas, pasta, and crackers

Legumes (bagged or canned): Chickpeas, black beans, white beans, lentils, kidney beans

Fish: Salmon, sardines, tuna (fresh, canned, or packaged)

Oils: Extra-virgin olive, canola, grape-seed, sesame, avocado

Vinegars: Balsamic, apple cider, flavored vinegars

Spices and herbs: Turmeric, black pepper, oregano, cinnamon, ginger, garlic, peppermint, parsley, rosemary, sage

Nuts and nut butters: Peanuts, almonds, walnuts, Brazil nuts, cashews, pistachios, pecans, pine nuts

Coffee and tea

Must-have refrigerator items

Vegetables for the week: Asparagus, beets, broccoli, Brussels sprouts, carrots, cauliflower, butternut and spaghetti squash, carrots, dark leafy greens, kale, onions, zucchini, red and yellow peppers, and other favorites

Fruits for the week: Apples, pears, berries (blueberries, blackberries, raspberries, strawberries), grapefruit, oranges, lemon, kiwifruit, melons, grapes, pineapple, bananas

Soup ingredients: Low-sodium vegetable broth and chicken broth, stewed tomatoes, legumes, frozen vegetables

Eggs and dairy: Eggs, part-skim cheeses, Parmesan cheese, fat-free or low-fat Greek yogurt, low-fat or fat-free milk and unsweetened milk swaps (almond, cashew, oat, hemp)

Condiments: Mustard, sauerkraut, salsa

Salad enhancers: Hearts of palm, water chestnuts, artichokes, roasted peppers

Lunch meats: Turkey with no preservatives or nitrates added

Must-have freezer items

Frozen fruits and vegetables: Assorted, without added sauces

Fish: Wild salmon, flounder, branzino, red snapper, tuna, cod

Poultry: Chicken breasts (on the bone, boneless, skinless), lean ground turkey or chicken, whole chicken

Meat: Lean ground beef, lean cuts of steak (sirloin, eye of round, bottom round)

Meatless burgers: Veggie burgers, bean burgers

 Avoid the crowds by shopping on a Wednesday. For some real solitude, hit the aisles after 9:00 p.m.

Shop till you drop

I won't ever ask you to change where you shop, but I'd like to open your eyes to how. Heeding these research-based guidelines can save you time, money, and calories:

Shop with something in your belly. If you are hungry, you may be tempted to buy junk food and nibble along the way or bring it home.

Shop with your list and stick to it. I like to keep the list on my phone. If you're at all like me, you may accidentally leave your paper list at home or in the car. Pick the method that works best for you.

Shop the perimeter of the store. Most prepackaged foods are in the center aisles, and you want the fresh foods. Wind your way around each of the produce aisles.[3]

Always check the label. In a National Institutes of Health study, researchers discovered that cereal wrapped in wholesome-looking packaging can be less healthy than cereal that screams sugar. Case in point: Overall, Kellogg's healthy-sounding Cracklin' Oat Bran had more sugar and calories and fewer nutrients than the colorful, artificially flavored Kellogg's Froot Loops. Froot Loops cereal is hardly health food.[4]

Focus on shopping and making smart choices. Multitasking makes you 40 percent less productive, so don't text and shop.[5]

Buy small. Researchers from KU Leuven in Belgium determined that the bigger the package, the more children (just like adults) will eat, *especially if the product is sugary.*[6] If you have young children who are pulling boxes off the shelf as you stroll the aisles, buy the smallest package, turn the trip into a teachable moment about healthy food choices, or shop without your little love bugs.

Use the self-checkout lane. Women are 32 percent and men 16.7 percent less likely to fall prey to impulse purchases such as candy when they're busy checking out. A whopping 80 percent of candy purchases are impulse buys![7]

For those of you who prefer to grocery shop online, the same rules apply.

When shopping, take note: Dr. Pierre Chandon, a marketing professor at the business school INSEAD, found that shoppers are generally good at being able to tell when a product is downsized. In fact, they are quick to complain! However, the reverse doesn't hold true. We have a hard time being able to tell whether our favorite food packages got bigger, and therefore we may eat more than we realize.[8]

 Bring your water bottle with you when you shop. Quenching your thirst can keep you full and less prone to wanting what's not on your list. You'll also have the occasion to get in a glass or two of water.

Whatever you bring into your kitchen you will eat. Shopping with intention puts healthy choices at your fingertips at home. And when hunger strikes, you'll have filling, nutritious foods at the ready. You'll always be prepared—now, that's what I call shopping like a chef!

Wedge of Wisdom

When Janet started eating a healthy snack an hour before grocery shopping, she was no longer tempted to head down the cookie aisle, which in the past she couldn't seem to resist. This small change— shopping with something in her stomach—made all the difference in her resolve to keep binge foods out of the house.

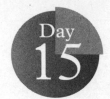

Dine Out Defensively

> One cannot think well, love well, sleep well, if one has not dined well.
>
> —Virginia Woolf

Americans love to eat out. Most of us spend more than half of our food budget on meals prepared outside the home.[1] Dining out also puts a dent in our calorie budget. As discussed in the "Gaining Weight? It's Your Portions!" chapter, you know that it's possible to consume upward of 2,000 calories (an entire day's worth!) in just one restaurant meal. When eating out, we're at the mercy of the restaurant, where meals are usually higher in calories, fat, salt, and sugar than home-cooked meals and where portions can be extra-large.[2] To lose weight or maintain weight loss, you don't have to give up eating out. You just have to wise up to your environment and dine out defensively.

Here are my top tips for dining out healthfully.

Bite-Sized Goodie Even child-sized restaurant meals are too big. Research conducted by the RAND Corporation reviewing portion sizes of kids' meals at chain restaurants found that à la carte items averaged 147 percent more calories than recommended by an expert panel. The panel determined that a kid's meal should contain no more than 600 calories (which includes 300 for the entrée, 100 for fried potatoes, and 150 for vegetables and salads), yet hundreds of meals exceeded this limit.[3]

Before you get there

Be prepared.

- Most restaurants display their menu online. Take a few minutes to look at it beforehand—not when you're hungry but after you've had a meal or a snack. Decide on something healthy and stick to it. Look for menu items that are baked, grilled, or roasted. Choose red sauce over cream sauce.
- Make a reservation so you don't have to wait in the bar or reach the point where you're famished.
- If you don't have time to view the menu in advance and you know the type of cuisine you will eat, plan accordingly. For example, if you're going Italian and you want to order pasta, don't have a sandwich for lunch.

Fill up before you head out. I try to eat something before I go out to eat. It prevents me from attacking the bread basket because I'm overhungry. A couple of hours before I'm scheduled to dine, I try to have a vegetable soup (homemade whenever possible), veggies and hummus, avocado and crackers, a low-sodium V8 juice, or a yogurt and fruit. I also carry around a small baggie filled with an ounce (a palm full) of nuts when I'm on the go. These snacks hit the spot but don't ruin my appetite. I still want to eat when I'm at the restaurant, but I'm able to stay mindful and make the best choices.

Drink water. Drink water before you go to the restaurant and when you're there. It helps to fill you up. And oftentimes, we think we are hungry when we are just thirsty.

Dress up! Make dining out a treat in and of itself by dressing up. Feeling elegant can also make you feel like eating less. And if you wear form-fitting clothes (not too tight) or a belt, you may be less tempted to overeat.

Take a lap around a buffet before you decide what to eat. Fill half your plate with veggies and pick one type of starch and one or two protein options. Most of your plate should have healthy food, with room for a little something fun.

Some restaurants focus on promoting healthy meals and vegetable dishes, but this can backfire because some people perceive healthy foods as less tasty. Stanford University researchers found that when the menu features exciting and indulgent descriptors of healthy foods (such as twisted carrots and dynamite beets), diners are all in.[4]

In 2018, as part of the menu labeling rule of the Affordable Care Act, the FDA is requiring chain restaurants with twenty or more locations, as well as grocery and convenience stores, to print nutrition information on their menus.[5] The driving factors: More people are eating out more often, and restaurant-goers want to make informed choices for weight and health matters.

Rule It Out

Once you have a meal's nutrition information, what do you do with it? Before ordering, compare different items and see which gives you the best bang for your (health) buck, and keep portion size in mind.

When ordering

Start your meal off right. It's better to fill up on a healthy salad or a vegetable or bean soup than bread and butter or chips. Or order a healthy appetizer such as grilled vegetables or artichoke. And remember to drink water or sparkling water.

Mind your portions. We can't change the size of a restaurant portion, but we can determine how we react to it. Great ways to avoid eating an entire oversized portion are to:

- Split an entrée with your dining partner. Don't concern yourself with surcharges for an extra plate. Focus on doing the right thing for you.
- Replate your plate by sharing different dishes. I do this all the time. I order a vegetarian dish loaded with veggies and my dining partner orders chicken or fish and then we split it up. Works like a charm.
- When you place your order, ask for a to-go carton at the same time. When you wrap up excess food right off the bat, you won't overeat and you will have an extra meal for later.
- Many entrées have it backward. They come with a large piece of meat and a small portion of veggies. Ask the server whether you can order extra vegetables, even if it costs more. Then wrap up half your meat portion.
- Steer clear of meals described with these words—jumbo, big, double, oversized. It means you are getting too much!
- Always order salad dressing on the side.
- Opt for whole grains (brown rice pilaf, quinoa, wild rice, whole-wheat pasta) instead of refined grains (white rice and pasta). Or order double veggies if you've had enough starch for the day.

- If given the choice, order a reduced-portion entrée or make a meal out of an appetizer and a side salad or other vegetables.
- Enjoy your company, eat slowly, and savor each bite.

Bite-Sized Goodie University of Minnesota researchers found that when people selected a reduced-sized entrée (a half sandwich instead of a full or a small salad instead of a large, for instance) in a restaurant or work-site setting, they consumed fewer calories and also wasted less food.[6] Another study found that when diners were invited to downsize their portion of Chinese food, up to 30 percent accepted the offer, and those who did saved 200 calories.[7]

When eating

Be mindful when eating.

- Chew your food completely before picking your fork up again. This gives you time to notice when you are getting full.
- Dress your salad by using the fork method—order your dressing on the side, dip your fork into the salad dressing, and then fill the dipped fork with salad. You'll use less salad dressing but still taste the flavor.

Slice of Advice When it comes to alcohol, think *one*. One drink on occasion is fine for most people. Drink more and we tend to eat more too, as alcohol lowers inhibitions and can make us hungry. Before ordering that second drink, have a glass of sparkling water, a glass of water with lemon, or a cup of herbal tea.

When finished

Cover it up. When you feel satisfied, cover your plate with your napkin and push it to the side. It's easy to nibble at what's left on your plate, but you don't have to finish your meal. Opt to feel good after eating rather than stuffed.

Skip or split the dessert. If you think you might want dessert, plan for it, share it, and don't feel guilty. Some restaurant desserts

GO HALFSIES

More than 50 percent of us eat a sandwich for lunch, but huge portions of refined bread, sauce, and processed meat can rack up the calories. University of Illinois researchers found that on the days we eat sandwiches we add an extra 100 calories, 7 grams of fat, 268 grams of sodium, and 3 grams of sugar to our daily intake. We also eat fewer fruits and vegetables on those days.[8] But sandwiches are so easy, quick, available, and tasty that no one wants to give them up. When I'm asked what kind of sandwich isn't fattening, I answer, "A half a sandwich." Make your sandwiches healthy and portion ready by following these tips to build a better sandwich:

- Choose a whole-grain bread or bun.
- Go easy on the cold cuts, skip the cheese, and choose a lean protein such as grilled fish, chicken, or turkey breast.
- Make it vegetarian: Swap the hamburger for a veggie burger or order a sandwich with tofu, tempeh, hummus, or white beans.
- Deli sandwiches can contain a pound of meat, so keep portions in mind. Share a whole sandwich, order half a sandwich, or wrap up the second half.
- Go topless and take off the top piece of bread.
- Always ask for veggies, which add nutrients and volume. Try dark lettuce, tomato, shredded carrot, peppers, and more.
- Order the topping on the side. Condiments tend to be high in sodium, and a little can go a long way. Ask for your sandwich dry, with the mayo or other sauces on the side, and use only what you need.

have more calories than the entrées. Unless it's a special occasion, skip dessert or have something light waiting for you at home. If you do order dessert, split it. Or ask for fruit (fruit isn't always on the menu, but many restaurants have it on hand) and a biscotto. Another option is to have something like sorbet, frozen yogurt, or a piece of your favorite chocolate waiting at home so you avoid caving in to ordering the double-dark-chocolate lava brownie with whipped cream.

Salad smarts

Salads as lunch or dinner entrées and salad bars are popular. But be careful. Salads can have more calories than a sandwich, so it helps to get some salad smarts.

Make sure your salad has the following:

- Bursts of different colors
- One protein choice—chicken, turkey, fish, eggs, legumes, tofu, tempeh
- An olive oil–based dressing, on the side (use a shot glass's worth—1–2 tablespoons, not more)
- Vinegar and fresh lemon, if you want (these are freebies!)
- One boost—avocado, olives, nuts, seeds, or cheese

Skip these items:

- Croutons, sesame sticks, and other similar toppings
- Caramelized nuts
- High-sugar dried fruit, such as dried cranberries
- Marinated vegetables, unless you use them as your dressing

Typical restaurant portions

We already know that portion sizes in restaurants are huge. But just how big are we talking? Take a look at this table, which shows you

Food	Typical portion size	Number of servings per food group
Chicken, fish, or beef entrée	6–9 ounces cooked	2–3 Meats
Cooked vegetable, side dish	1 cup	2 Vegetables
Rice or cooked grains, side dish	1 cup	2 Starches
Cheese pizza (personal pie)	3 ounces dough	3 Starches
	2–3 ounces cheese	2 Dairy
	½ cup tomato sauce	1 Vegetable
	Olive oil, 1–2 tablespoons	1–2 Fats
Pasta with marinara sauce (entrée)	3–4 cups pasta	6–8 Starches
	½–1 cup marinara sauce	1–2 Vegetables
Burrito	Tortilla, 2 ounces	2 Starches
	½ cup rice	1 Starch
	½ cup beans	1 Meat alternative
	3 ounces beef or chicken	1 Meat
	1–2 ounces cheese	1 Dairy
	½ cup salad	½ Vegetable
	¼ cup guacamole	1 Fat
	Sour cream, 2–3 tablespoons	1 Fat
Sushi, 1 roll (about 6 pieces)	½–1 cup rice	1–2 Starches
	Fish—varies by type of roll	½–1 Meat
	Vegetables, varies	½ Vegetable
	Avocado, 2 tablespoons	½ Fat
	Spicy roll containing mayonnaise, 1 tablespoon	1 Fat

the typical portion sizes and the number of servings per food group for a few sample meals. Restaurant portions are not universal, but this guide will help you to approximate.

It doesn't matter how much the restaurant serves you. It matters how much you actually eat!

Make any cuisine healthy

Here are several simple swaps you can make for some favorite cuisines.

American.
Start with a house salad with dressing on the side instead of a Caesar salad.
Order grilled instead of fried chicken or fish entrées.
Choose a baked potato instead of French fries.
Order steamed or sautéed vegetables instead of potatoes in gravy.
Order a veggie burger instead of a cheeseburger.

Chinese.
Choose steamed instead of fried dumplings.
Order steamed brown rice instead of fried rice and stick to a 1-cup portion.
Order entrées steamed or lightly sautéed, instead of fried.
Instead of spareribs, choose steamed or sautéed chicken with vegetables.
Order your favorite sauce on the side.

Italian.
Order pasta primavera instead of fettuccine alfredo.
Skip the extra cheese.
Order pasta in olive oil or tomato sauce instead of cream sauce and vodka sauce.

Start with a salad instead of fried mozzarella sticks.

Choose whole-wheat pastas whenever possible.

Mexican.

Start with gazpacho instead of nachos with cheese.

Order grilled fish or chicken instead of fried beef.

Choose baked beans and rice instead of refried beans.

When making a burrito, choose extra lettuce and tomato instead of extra cheese.

Choose salsa and guacamole instead of sour cream.

Japanese.

Start with a seaweed salad instead of fried bean curd.

Order steamed vegetables instead of vegetables tempura (battered and fried veggies).

Order sushi or sashimi instead of shrimp tempura.

Skip the spicy sauce.

French.

Start with a mixed green salad instead of French onion soup.

Order entrées in a wine-based sauce instead of béarnaise sauce.

Order lightly sautéed vegetables instead of creamy au gratin vegetables or potatoes.

Choose poached pears instead of crème caramel.

To lose weight, you don't need to abandon your favorite restaurants. The key to dining out defensively is being prepared and learning to pick the healthiest choices wherever you are, whether a buffet or a four-star French restaurant.

Wedge of Wisdom

Mary, a busy New York executive, eats out for most meals, for work
and pleasure. She put on some weight as her life revolved around
food eaten away from home. We came up with a few go-to meals
that she can order anywhere—grilled fish or chicken with vegetables
and a sweet potato, and a house salad to start, with dressing on the
side. She used this strategy a few times a week, and her weight-loss
efforts began to work. While I do not recommend it, you can eat out
most meals and still lose weight, if you plan correctly.

STAGE 3
Your Habits

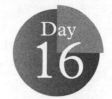

Be Your Own General

What you do today can improve all your tomorrows.

—Ralph Marston

A healthy lifestyle doesn't just happen. Eating on the fly and saying you'll exercise if you have time don't cut it. You need to plan to eat well and exercise just as you would plan for an important meeting or a trip. Like a four-star general, you need to take charge. And you need a good battle plan.

Planning for weight loss gives you structure, and structure gives you some level of predictability so you can plan ahead—key factors in making it happen. While it takes time to create a schedule, it saves time in the long run, keeps you on track, and most definitely reduces stress. If you know what you're packing for lunch tomorrow, you can ensure you have the ingredients on hand and make it the night before. The alternative is to frantically search the fridge at 7:00 a.m. for food you don't have and run out the door empty-handed to avoid being late for work.

People who plan their meals and cook at home have healthier diets (with more fruits and veggies) and less obesity, save money, and avoid frequent stops at fast-food restaurants,[1] all of which spells weight loss.

Plan to bring your lunch to work at least a few days a week so you're certain to eat healthy, portion-ready meals.

Your weight-loss battle plan

Let's look at what goes into an ironclad weight-loss battle plan.

Plan what you'll eat for the day, and when. The prediary (Day #2: Write It before You Bite It, page 56) is your best offense. At least a day or two ahead of time, write down what you will eat. This gives you time to think it through. I know that before you began this program you probably had no idea what your next meal would be, but I encourage you to give tomorrow's meals a thought, as best you can.

Cook for the week. To really get ahead of the game, set an afternoon aside to prepare meals for the week and portion them out accordingly. (See Day #10: Cook Like a Portion Pro, page 111).

Plan your exercise. You know the drill: Before starting an exercise routine, check with your doctor. Then, consider what activities best suit you. You might want to join a health club, work out with a fitness trainer, attend classes, buy a bicycle, or walk to school or work. Decide when you will exercise and for how long. I recommend you exercise for at least 30 minutes four to five days a week. If you are exercising after work, you may want to pack a gym bag and bring it along with you so you don't have to stop at home, where you might get busy or tired and talk yourself out of going. (Check out Day #24: Step It Up, page 209, for more on exercise.)

Put it on the calendar. Lunch at noon; yoga, Tuesday at 5:30 p.m.; weight lifting, Wednesday at 5:30 p.m.; grocery shopping, Wednesday at 9:00 p.m. Be specific and just do it. Putting it on the calendar makes it a priority. And you consider it done!

Applaud a job well done. Encourage yourself to keep doing

what you're doing by rewarding yourself (not with food!) for practicing your new habits.

Bite-Sized Goodie Planning your meals ahead of time may help with weight loss. University of Bristol researchers learned that overweight individuals are less likely to take into account what they already ate when considering their next meal. In other words, they are more likely to eat on the fly.[2]

Old habits don't have to die hard

Chances are, your plan includes some new routines—perhaps exercising regularly or drinking more water—that will require you to develop new habits. When you ring in the new, it's out with the old. We've all got eating patterns and idiosyncrasies. Some habits serve us and some don't. But make no mistake about it: Eating is a behavior, and your habits determine your behavior. So taking some time to look at your food habits can lead to a weight-loss breakthrough.

Breaking an old habit isn't as hard as you might think. Sometimes you just need to replace it with something new and better, do it consistently, and watch for the domino effect.

Slice of Advice If you're in the habit of pouring your cereal into your bowl before you pour the milk, keep it up. Researchers from the University of Hohenheim in Germany found that people who poured the milk first gave themselves larger portions of milk and cereal.[3]

For an effortless transition from old to new, support yourself in your new habits. As best-selling author Gretchen Rubin writes in *Better Than Before*, you can strengthen good habits by making them more convenient.[4] Keep a bowl of fruit on the counter, stock your fridge and cupboards with healthy foods, purchase a few portion props to help you get a handle on your food portions, and keep a packed gym bag in the car. And you can squash a bad habit by making it inconvenient. Get rid of junk food, and store treats on shelves you need the stepladder to reach.

Rubin also suggests that you know yourself well enough that you can shape a habit to suit you. Looking over your Portion Tracker is a great start. Do you notice you eat more when stressed, during a certain time of day, or when around certain people? The next step is finding new habits to crowd out the old ones. Try on some changes, see how they fit, and before long what feel like temporary, even awkward, changes will become natural and permanent.

Begin to develop good habits as soon as you start the Program. You are starting fresh, with a clean slate. The habits we set up early on tend to remain with us.

Make the shift

Here are some common habits some of us could stand to lose. If any sound familiar, break them by bringing in something new.

Let it go: I feel like I am giving up so much.
Bring it in: Be positive.

For the best chance at success, focus on what you can do and have—not on what you're giving up. Instead of dwelling on not eating sugar, focus on the fact that you get to eat a lot of sweet-tasting fruit—and how good you'll feel as the pounds start to drop.

Let it go: I come home from work famished.
Bring it in: Eat a satisfying snack 2 hours before leaving work.

Include fruits or veggies along with some protein. Bring fruit and a cheese stick as a snack; carry a small bag of nuts; keep baby carrots and cut-up veggies in the fridge. Be prepared. Don't stop at the convenience or grocery store when you're starving. When you go home or to the gym with something in your stomach, you will make healthier food choices the rest of the day.

Let it go: I stop at the same coffee shop every morning and order a bagel with cream cheese and a mocha topped off with whipped cream.
Bring it in: Order tea or coffee with low-fat milk and a veggie omelet with a slice of whole-grain toast.

Or eat breakfast at home, pack fruit and yogurt to go, and take a different route to work.

Let it go: I give up easily.
Bring it in: Think about the areas of your life where you're a fighter and you don't give up.

You might be a superstar parent but be passive with your health and lifestyle. It's up to you to decide what's worth fighting for. If you want to lose weight and feel great, summon your fighting spirit—the one you rely on to be successful in other areas of life.

Let it go: I'm a stress eater.
Bring it in: Sit for a few moments with your urge to run to the kitchen.

If it doesn't pass, have cut-up fruits and veggies at the ready. They're on the Plan. They're freebies. They'll satisfy your desire to eat. And you won't get fat from eating them. Or call a pal and get outside and take a walk. Changing your environment and meeting up with a close friend can help you de-stress.

Let it go: I hate wasting food. I remember my grandmother's mantra: "There are people in the world who are starving... Finish your food!"
Bring it in: Pack it up.

I wouldn't call a reluctance to waste food a bad habit, but it could get in the way of weight loss if it interferes with portion control.

If you feel you have to finish everything on your plate or you can't get yourself to throw out perfectly fine (albeit unhealthy) food stored in your cupboards, get in the habit of packing it up. Portion out chips and candy in snack-size baggies. Freeze leftovers in single or double portions, depending on how many people you typically serve. If it's a question of eat it or waste it, wrap it up. Or consider donating unopened canned or dry goods to your local food bank.

Let it go: I can't seem to stick to an exercise routine.
Bring it in: Don't think about it. As the Nike ad says, "Just do it!"

Stick to your word when it comes to exercising. Put it in your Portion Tracker or on your calendar. Look at the clock and go. Giving into excuses is easy—we can talk ourselves out of almost anything. You don't have to run a marathon. You just need 30 or 45 minutes of your day. Some days we really don't feel up to a workout or have a genuine excuse. Allow yourself that. But if excuses start to rule, conjure up the leader in you. Generals don't announce a strong battle plan and then talk themselves out of it. They follow through, rain or shine.

Let it go: I get absorbed in my work and skip meals.
Bring it in: Do your best to eat structured meals and snacks.

Ohio State University researchers found that skipping meals promotes gorging behavior and abdominal fat in mice.[5] It may do the same to us humans. When we skip meals, we tend to compensate by overeating later. Schedule a time to eat. Eat something, even if it's a snack. Be mindful. Stay structured. It's probably one of the best things you can do for your weight-loss efforts.

Let it go: Once I start losing weight, I celebrate by telling myself I can eat more.
Bring it in: Set up a healthy reward system for yourself.

For instance, set a mini-goal and then give yourself a nonfood reward when you reach it. Buy the new watch you've been eyeing or order theater tickets. Set up rewards along the way to keep yourself motivated.

Let it go: I cave in to eating treats when others insist I have some.
Bring it in: Protecting your health and goals is not rude.

You don't need to pretend you're one of those people who can eat a chocolate cake and still be thin. When the food pushers insist, say, "No, thank you." Or just be honest and say you've been losing weight and you want to stick to your plan.

 Take some quiet time and write down five habits you'd like to change. What new habits can you replace them with? Write them in your journal or on your Portion Tracker. Put them on your calendar. And do them.

Generals expect to meet their goals—everything they do is with victory in mind. Give yourself some marching orders, stick to them, soldier on, and put on your armor when pressured by outside forces. *Own* your goals. From now on, you're a four-star general in a war against oversized portions.

Wedge of Wisdom

Marcy, a twenty-eight-year-old busy mom who also freelances, ate many of her meals and snacks on the fly. She also felt too busy to keep a record of her food intake, so she had no idea what—and how much—she was actually eating. When she came to see me, we set up a structure for her eating program. She started planning meals in advance and using the Portion Tracker. These tactics (as opposed to having to starve!) worked and helped her lose those stubborn 15 pounds she'd been carrying.

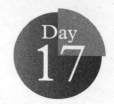

Eat Mindfully

Mindful eating is a way to become reacquainted with the
guidance of our internal nutritionist.

—Jan Chozen Bays

Mindfulness is the practice of focusing your attention on the present
moment. It's kind of like meditation in motion. You make yourself
mindful of whatever you are doing, whether chopping vegetables or
sitting on the subway. As you wash your hands, for instance, you
feel the water, note the temperature, and relish how the water and
soap feel against your skin. You're not thinking about the meeting you just got out of or the fact that you need to walk the dog
when you get home. Mindfulness is about presence and acceptance.
You accept all your feelings and thoughts in this moment without
judgment.

When we apply mindfulness to eating, we're fully tuned in to
our appetite, appreciate our food, note when we are satisfied, avoid
eating impulsively, and can lose weight as a result. In an Oregon
Research Institute study, participants who practiced mindful eating
for six weeks lost on average 9 pounds during the study and beyond.[1]
Over the course of a six-month mindfulness seminar, participants
in a University of Wisconsin study lost on average 27 pounds and
did not gain it back in the three months following the seminar.[2]

The positive effects of mindfulness also extend to eating behaviors related to weight gain. McGill University researchers analyzed data from nineteen studies with 1,160 participants examining the effects of mindfulness-based interventions on weight loss and found that the interventions helped with weight loss as well as emotional eating, binge eating, and anxiety.[3] For overweight adolescents and adults, mindfulness led to more self-control and reduced impulsive food choices.[4]

Mindfulness can also prevent weight gain. Researchers at North Carolina State University reviewed the literature on mindful eating and found that the strategy helps with food cravings and portion control. Study participants had greater awareness of their bodies, were tuned in to hunger signals, and had more self-compassion to boot.[5] Lastly, researchers at the University of Liverpool found that when people ate lunch attentively, they ate 30 percent less later in the day.[6]

Researchers at the University of Rhode Island learned that setting aside enough time to eat, rather than gulping your meals down on the go or at your desk, can help you lose weight. During the study, the women who ate slowly felt fuller with less food and drank more water than those who ate quickly.[7] Texas Christian University researchers found similar results: People who took 22 minutes instead of 9 minutes to eat consumed up to 88 fewer calories.[8]

How to be present for your meal

Being mindful when you eat is simple. When you're ready to eat, whether a snack or a full-fledged meal, do the following to help keep you in the moment:

Sit down. This is a pet peeve of mine. I see so many people at events who grab food from a buffet and carry around a plate, walking, talking, and eating. They aren't paying attention to what they are eating, let alone how much. Thoughtfully fill up a plate, sit down to eat, and savor each bite so you actually remember the experience.

Savor every bite. Cut your food into bite-sized pieces and chew slowly and thoroughly. Chewing releases flavor, so the longer you chew, the more you taste your food. Notice the textures and smell. This act alone reduces how many calories you consume because you feel more satisfied. It also improves digestion and allows your body to absorb more nutrients than if you inhale your food.[9]

Set it down. Put your eating utensil down between bites. Chew your food without preparing the next forkful. When you're done with one bite, pause to drink water, talk, or assess how full you are, and then approach your next bite or decide you've had enough. And don't forget to breathe.

Unplug. Turn off or put away all electronic devices. Do not eat at your desk ("al desko"), in front of a computer, or while watching television. If you do, by the time you pause long enough to look at your plate, it will be empty. University of Bristol researchers found that people who played a computer game while eating ate faster, ate nearly twice as much, and felt less full than people who were not distracted while eating.[10]

Keep good company. Brazil's dietary guidelines are hailed as being among the best in the world. They focus on eating whole and minimally processed foods. They also emphasize eating with family, friends, or colleagues and getting everyone involved in cooking and cleaning up as a way to enjoy meals and feel more satisfied.[11] If you're with others, be mindful of the conversation. Enjoy the entire experience. When food and dining (and cleanup!) are pleasurable, you will feel more satisfied.

Renew your relationship with food. Eat only what you feel good about putting into your body. You might want to plant a vegetable garden, pick your own fruit at orchards or berry farms, bake your own bread, or visit farmers' markets more regularly. Be grateful and appreciate that you have healthy food to eat.

 Buy a pair of chopsticks. If you're not accustomed to eating with them, they will slow you down. Eating with chopsticks may also improve your mind-body connection.

Researchers at Kyushu University in Japan found that the faster a person eats, the more likely he or she will be overweight. Normal-speed eaters are 29 percent more likely to be obese than slow eaters. Fast eaters are 42 percent more likely to be obese.[12]

The Hunger Rater

Most of us have what I like to call a built-in Hunger Rater. It tells us when we're hungry and when we can stop eating. If we've been overeating for too long, our Hunger Rater is likely broken—we've lost the sense of how it feels to be hungry or satisfied. To get back in touch with your Hunger Rater, try being mindful of your true hunger signals. After a few days of eating thoughtful portions and being mindful, your Hunger Rater will be working better.

Use the following to rate your hunger:

1. Ravenous
2. Hungry
3. Neutral
4. Satisfied
5. Overfull

The best time to eat is when you're hungry (#2)—not when you're so famished that you're dizzy or irritable and not because

HARA HACHI BU

Before a meal, some people in Okinawa, Japan, recite the phrase *hara hachi bu*. It's a gentle reminder to stop eating when they are no longer hungry. What's the difference between being full and no longer being hungry? About 20 percent—and 20 minutes. People who practice *hara hachi bu* stay mindful enough to stop eating when they are about 80 percent full. This ancient practice gives the stomach the 20 minutes it needs to register that it is full. It's a natural way to sense portion control. For Okinawans it works. They consume fewer calories than the average American. And rates of heart disease, stroke, and cancer are up to 80 percent lower in Okinawa than they are in America.[13]

you're stressed or having a food craving. Healthy hunger is a slight pang that tells you it's time to eat. Ideally, you will finish eating when you're at #3 or #4, or about 75 or 80 percent full. This sensation usually happens when you first begin to think you've had enough. If you continue eating, you will soon start to feel overfull, or at #5.

Feeling satisfied after eating has more to do with the brain than the stomach. It takes a full 20 minutes for hormones in your intestines to signal to the brain that you've had enough. So, give your body the time it needs to do its job—be mindful. Either eat slowly or wait a full 20 minutes before heading for seconds.[14]

Wedge of Wisdom

My client Marty, a forty-one-year-old lawyer, used to eat while working because he didn't want to waste a minute. He had no idea what or how much he ate or whether he was full or still hungry. When he came to see me, I suggested he turn off autopilot. He found it hard at first but kept trying. He ate more slowly and paid attention to the act of eating. These habits, along with his food plan, helped him lose 35 pounds—and keep it off.

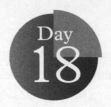

Swap and Drop

Diets are for those who are thick and tired of it.

—Mary Tyler Moore

Weight loss doesn't have to turn your life upside down. Small changes can go a long way. Swapping one food for a healthy, lower-calorie food while remaining true to your portions is one really easy way to supercharge your weight loss. Swapping is flexible, can help with your weight-loss efforts, and sometimes means you can eat more. You're not giving something up but trying something different. And while I don't want you stressing over exact calorie counts, some swaps can even reduce a calorie intake by half, which is like money in your weight-loss bank account.

Swaps are also about eating smarter and being healthier. Healthy beverage swaps such as drinking water or unsweetened tea and coffee instead of sugary drinks yields weight loss[1] and is associated with a lower risk of diabetes.[2] Choosing whole grains instead of refined wheat has been shown to decrease the percentage of body fat and improve blood lipid profiles in postmenopausal women.[3]

When you know what to swap, you're more likely to do it. Researchers from Newcastle University in the UK who evaluated a campaign to get families to switch to lower-sugar and lower-fat items found that the campaign worked. Up to 32 percent of people

SWAPPORTUNITIES

So many different varieties of swaps exist. Start with the list in this chapter and then come up with some on your own. To help you remember the different kinds of swaps, I've come up with a mnemonic: SLIM.

SLIM

Size swaps: Swap from a larger size to a smaller one or from a double to a single.

Lean swaps: Swap higher-calorie choices for healthier foods within the same food group.

Ingenious swaps: Swap foods from one food group for foods in another group that are similar in taste and appearance, often higher in nutrients, and lower in calories.

More please swaps: Swap a smaller for a bigger portion.

purchased lower-sugar drinks, up to 24 percent chose lower-sugar cereal, and up to 58 percent swapped to a lower-fat dairy product.[4] So, in this chapter I'm going to share some "swapportunities."

S—Size swaps

By now, you know more than most about healthy portion sizes. And while I've steered you away from unhealthy foods, you might decide to have them on occasion. Size swapping can help you stick with your portions, even when driving through the fast-food lane. These swaps shave off not only calories but also sugar, fat, and sodium and are more in line with healthy portion sizes outlined in the Plan. Here are some size swaps that can save you more than 1,300 calories:

Order an appetizer portion of pasta instead of a main-dish portion. Many main-dish pasta portions contain at least 3 cups, an entire day's worth of starch. Appetizer portions contain about 1½ cups of pasta, enough for an entire meal. Ask for fresh tomato sauce and a large side of veggies, and your portion is far from skimpy. Switching from a main dish to an appetizer portion of pasta can save you at least 300 calories.

Order the small. (Note: In Starbucks, a small is called "tall.") Drinks contain calories, so go small. Switching from a Starbucks venti (20-ounce) Frappuccino to a tall (12-ounce) cup saves you around 170 calories. Downsize your smoothie, too. Many medium smoothies contain 20-plus ounces and 300–500 calories. A small (usually 12 or 16 ounces) is still big and may run 200–400 calories. A large store-bought smoothie can easily top 800 calories if you are not careful.

Go single, instead of double or triple. The fast-food industry is notorious for selling single, double, and triple hamburgers. If you're splurging on fast food, you don't have to choose the biggest size. Order the single instead of the double burger. McDonald's Grand Mac and Mac Jr., both introduced in 2017, are a case in point. The original Big Mac contains 540 calories. The Grand Mac (basically a double Big Mac!) contains 860 calories, while the Mac Jr. contains 460 calories. Go for the Mac Jr. and save 400 calories.

L—Lean swaps

Lean swaps are healthier, lower-calorie versions of some of your favorite foods within the same food group. To make a lean swap, pick your favorite food and look for alternatives in the same food group. Some examples of lean swaps include the following:

Choose whole fruit instead of juice. Juice tends to be high in sugar and low in fiber. Fresh fruit, on the other hand, contains more fiber than the juice and has a higher water content, both of which are excellent for weight loss. Eating an orange instead of guzzling down a pint of orange juice can save you more than 150 calories. Imagine how many calories you can save if you make this switch daily.

Opt for mashed avocado instead of mayonnaise. Avocado is a healthier fat than mayo and tastes great in egg or tuna salad or on a turkey sandwich.

Start your day with whole-grain cereal instead of a bran muffin. Muffins these days are oversized, often weighing in at 5–7 ounces, containing 5–7 starch servings and more than 500 calories! However, because it is just one item, and contains the healthy-sounding term "bran" in its name, we often overlook its high-calorie content. Switch to a cup of whole-grain cereal with a cup of low-fat milk or calcium-fortified almond milk and save at least 4 starch servings and around 300 calories. Or opt for oatmeal. When you make it yourself, you measure out your portion and know exactly how much goes into your bowl.

Choose grilled salmon steak over beefsteak. You'll get a dose of healthy omega-3 fatty acids, shown to reduce the risk of heart disease.[5]

Choose plant-based protein such as legumes instead of animal protein. Going meatless on more than just Mondays is good for your waist and your overall health.[6] Have a lentil stew or a tempeh and vegetable stir-fry with brown rice instead of a steak or lamb chops. Enjoy a black bean burger instead of a hamburger.

Choose skinless chicken breast over dark meat with the skin. You'll cut calories and, better yet, greatly reduce your intake of saturated fat. The skin on chicken does not have any redeeming qualities, so I suggest skipping it. If you are not a fan of skinless white meat, add some teriyaki sauce or barbecue sauce, or bake with panko crumbs.

Experiment with whole-grain sourdough bread or sprouted grains over white breads and even whole-grain breads.

Sourdough bread tends to be easier on the digestive tract. I've worked with many clients who thought they couldn't tolerate the gluten in bread, but they do well with sourdough bread. Breads made from sprouted grains taste similar to (or better than!) breads made from whole-grain flour, but your body may be able to better absorb nutrients from the sprouted grains.

Swap beef for bison. If you're cutting back on red meat but need a break from fish or chicken, try bison (buffalo) meat. Compared with 80 percent lean beef, bison contains less total fat and saturated fat and has a little more protein.

Slice of Advice

Love pizza and want to enjoy it? Here's a swapportunity—choose whole-wheat crust instead of white-flour crust. Pile on extra veggies. And swap that second slice for a green salad. Here are a size swap and a lean swap in action!

Bite-Sized Goodie

Eggs are "egg-cellent"—but choose scrambled eggs with veggies instead of a store-bought egg sandwich. I love making eggs with a generous helping of tomatoes, spinach, and mushrooms to boost fiber and nutrient intake and increase my portion exponentially.

I—Ingenious swaps

Ingenious swaps replace some of your favorite high-calorie food with food similar in taste and appearance. By making these swaps, you gain fiber and nutrients.

Starch swaps. If you're craving rice or pasta but have eaten all of your starches for the day, consider the following:

- Make pasta from spiraled zucchini or butternut squash, or try shirataki noodles (also called konnyaku noodles). These Asian noodles are made from konjac yams and have as little as 10–20 calories per cup as compared to 200 calories in a cup of cooked pasta.

- Make pizza with a cauliflower crust instead of wheat. You'll cut a lot more than gluten.
- Instead of pita chips, dip sliced peppers into your hummus or guacamole. You'll save calories and gain fiber and lots of vitamin C.
- Use grated cauliflower or celery root instead of rice or mashed potatoes to increase nonstarchy vegetable intake. You will save on starches and calories.
- Use walnuts, sunflower seeds, or roasted chickpeas in your salad instead of croutons. You may not save too many calories, but you will get the added health benefits of seeds and nuts.

Volume lovers, take note: A half cup of cooked pasta contains the same number of calories as 5 cups of zoodles!

M—More please swaps

Sometimes you want to eat more. These swaps are great for volume lovers.

Swap your raisins for grapes. Grow your fruit portion by switching from a small box (¼ cup) of raisins to a full cup of grapes. This swap goes for all dried fruit. Switch from dried apricots and figs to the fresh varieties.

Swap your glass of wine for a wine spritzer. Add a couple of ounces of wine to a glass of seltzer water and drink two.

Swap your breakfast cereal. Switch from a serving of granola (¼ cup) to a serving of ready-to-eat whole-grain oats (Cheerios, 1 cup) or puffed brown rice (2 cups) and eat more for fewer calories.

Add some berries and milk and you have a hearty portion. Add a tablespoon or two of crushed nuts or flaxseeds for some crunch and added nutrition.

Use water instead of oil. Steam vegetables and you can eat as many as you want without exceeding your fat budget. Cook and cleanup time are fast and easy. To save your fats for that avocado toast you've been craving, skimp on oil and poach instead of fry your eggs.

On the Plan, losing weight is not about deprivation. It's about eating smart. When presented with a choice, think in terms of what's better for you, and you'll be a professor of swaps before you know it.

Wedge of Wisdom

Cindy loved pasta. She didn't do very well with a small portion either. I suggested she get a tabletop spiralizer and experiment with spiraled veggies. She began to swap her pasta for spiraled veggies of all sorts—zucchini, beets, carrots, and butternut squash. She added olive oil, garlic, and Parmesan for a yummy meal. And her kids loved it too!

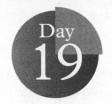

Power Up Your Snacks

I never worry about diets. The only carrots that interest me
are the number you get in a diamond.

—Mae West

In this chapter, I teach you how to snack smart, or turn to snacks
that power you up without adding unnecessary calories. A late
afternoon snack, especially, can energize you for an evening exercise
routine, fill you up so you don't crash at your desk, and tide you over
so you aren't ravenous before your next meal. A healthy snack may
even set you up to make better meal choices and stick to healthy
portion sizes.

Snacks aren't limited to freebies. Snack time is your time to get
creative and pair different food groups into light, satisfying refresh-
ments you can sink your teeth into. That doesn't mean chips and
dip, though!

The perfect pair

When it comes to snacks, you might try to get by with an apple or
just a palm full of nuts. But if you're still hungry, you scout out the
kitchen or your desk for more. When all you can find are nuts, you

end up overeating them and your healthy snack turns into a high-calorie diversion. That's what I'd call a "snaccident." We definitely want to avoid that.

When it comes to feeling satisfied, the best snacks pair a fruit, veggie, or whole grain with a protein or a fat. These combinations create satisfying snacks—they're nourishing and energizing and keep you full longer than a single-food-group snack. Combinations also taste good and beat a dry rice cake by a long shot. Appendix B (page 259) includes an extensive list of healthy (and fun!) snacks. Following are some ideas to get you started:

- Apple with 2 teaspoons peanut, almond, or cashew butter
- Avocado toast—¼ avocado on a slice of whole-grain toast or crackers (1 ounce) or 2 rice cakes
- Blueberries and strawberries with ½ cup cottage cheese topped with 1–2 tablespoons slivered almonds
- Crispbread (1 ounce) with tomato and feta cheese (about ¼ cup)
- Frozen mixed berries or fresh melon topped with 2 tablespoons crushed walnuts
- Hard-boiled egg and mixed veggies (red peppers, celery, and carrots)
- Homemade kale or beet chips
- Low-fat Greek yogurt with blackberries and 1 tablespoon walnuts
- Low-sodium V8 juice and a part-skim mozzarella cheese stick with 1 ounce whole-grain crackers
- Mixed vegetables (jicama, carrots, cucumbers) with ¼ cup hummus
- Mug of vegetable, split pea, or lentil soup
- Packaged tuna (2–3 ounces) with whole-grain crackers (1 ounce)
- Peanut butter (1 tablespoon) on a rice cake
- Roasted chickpeas or edamame and sliced red and yellow peppers and cherry tomatoes

- Smoothie—½ cup blueberries, ½ apple, ½ cup greens, with 1 cup unsweetened vanilla almond milk, fat-free milk, or cold water, and ½–1 cup crushed ice (or 4–6 ice cubes)
- Whole-grain crackers (1 ounce) with 1 tablespoon almond butter or 1 ounce cheese
- Whole-wheat pita bread (1 ounce) with cucumbers, tomatoes, and ¼ cup hummus
- Lettuce wrap with sliced turkey (2 ounces), sliced apple, and mustard

Need a healthy crunch? Mix 2 cups popcorn (a whole grain!) with a handful of nuts and seasoning. Or make a healthy trail mix by combining ½ cup whole-grain cereal (Cheerios or Barbara's Puffins), ¼ cup roasted chickpeas, 2 tablespoons of your favorite nuts and seeds, and 1 tablespoon dried blueberries or cherries for a sweet taste.

To snack or not to snack?

But when is snack time, exactly? For many people, snack time has morphed into a day of grazing. More and more people are eating around their schedules, rather than scheduling their lives around traditional mealtimes. We are eating more calories from snacks than we were in the past, which can be linked to weight gain, as our snacking habits may be adding unnecessary calories.[1] Half the time, what we put in our mouth is a snack, as opposed to a meal. Ninety percent of people snack throughout the day, and close to 10 percent of these snackers have replaced all three meals with snacks![2]

Turning snacking into an all-day affair encourages mindless nibbling. You most likely consume extra calories but feel as if you haven't really eaten. It's too easy to forget what and how much you ate. You're better off eating structured meals with a midafternoon and an after-dinner snack, if needed. You know yourself best and when you are hungriest, so it is ultimately up to you to decide when to snack.

Slice of Advice Nosh on whole foods that put you to work and you'll eat less. When you have to peel or shell a food, the rate at which you eat naturally slows down. Whole foods that make you work include oranges, grapefruit, pomegranate, and edamame in their shells. Shell nuts (pistachios, walnuts, almonds, and filberts) yourself; just seeing the pile of empty shells is enough to make you want to stop.

Are you prone to snaccidents?

Pay attention when you snack, and you'll be better able to keep your portions in line. One cup of store-bought trail mix, for instance, can have upward of 700 calories. If you're snacking and watching television at the same time, you might eat 1 cup or the entire bag of trail mix in one sitting without realizing it.

I encourage you to assemble healthy, portion-ready snacks at home. Buying portion-ready snacks is also an option—and it might help you eat less. Researchers at the University of Tennessee–Knoxville found that overweight people ate fewer pretzels when eating from a single-serve package as opposed to a large bag.[3]

Bite-Sized Goodie Give your snack as much attention as you would give your meal and you might eat less. In a recent study, researchers at the University of Surrey in the UK found that people ate "significantly more" sweet treats after eating a bowl of pasta labeled as a snack compared to people given the same amount of pasta labeled as a meal. One reason why participants who ate the snack pasta ate more sweets afterward may be that they ate standing up and used plastic bowls and spoons. The others ate their pasta off a ceramic plate, used metal utensils, and sat down at a table to eat.[4] Sit down and treat yourself well!

Treat time

Craving something fun? That's why I allow treats. Treats and sweets are not a food group, so you don't need them for good health. Sometimes, you might just want one. You're allowed up to two treats a day, but shoot for zero to one. Save it for when you really want it so it feels like a treat. These are the snacks you want to plan for so they feel legal. My clients tend to do best when they plan a treat for after dinner—a fudge pop, a small frozen yogurt, or ½ cup ice cream.

Here are some fun DIY snacks to enjoy after dinner that won't break your calorie budget. See Appendix B for more delicious ideas.

- Banana peanut butter "ice cream," made with just ripe bananas and peanut butter
- Baked cinnamon apple chips
- Very berry frozen ice pop, made with blended berries, unsweetened vanilla almond milk, 2 teaspoons peanut butter powder, and crushed ice
- Oversized strawberries dipped in 2–3 teaspoons almond butter and 1 tablespoon cocoa chips or cocoa powder; eat hot (warm in the microwave for 30 seconds) or cold (freeze for 30 minutes prior to eating)

Slice of Advice Shy away from eating chocolate or yogurt-coated protein, energy, or granola bars. People like them because they consider them to be healthy grab 'n' go snacks. Some of these bars, however, have nearly as many calories as a candy bar and are high in sugar. And there's really no yogurt in the yogurt-covered bars.

How to break the midnight munchie habit

An American Heart Association study linked late-night snacking and obesity[5]—in part because people tend to snack on unhealthy foods such as chips and candy, and we don't burn off much of what we eat before we hit the hay. If you're in the habit of eating late at night, ease into a new pattern by trying these tips:

- Plan a healthy, portion-ready snack.
- Eat it at the table, sitting down (not in front of the television set or computer).
- Replace chips or another treat snack with something healthy, such as berries, a baked apple, or an orange. Or try kale, beet, or carrot chips.
- Have a cup of hot herbal tea. With so many flavors to choose from these days, you can have a sweet flavor (vanilla almond), a savory choice (turmeric ginger), or a calming blend (lavender chamomile).
- Give yourself time for the food craving to pass: Think of two or three things you can do instead of eat. Take a warm bath, knit, or call a friend.

Make a portion-perfect nut case: Put ¼ cup nuts in a small tin or a mini-container. Be sure it is lightweight and secure so you can take it with you wherever you go.

Supersize your snack!

Sometimes you just want more! And you don't just want a piece of fruit or steamed vegetables. Try these options when you need something more:

- 3 cups air-popped popcorn topped with Parmesan cheese
- Spaghetti squash dusted with cinnamon
- Baked carrot and zucchini fries
- Roasted cauliflower. One of my clients was a chef. For a healthy snack, she roasted a whole cauliflower with her favorite herbs

and spices, a little olive oil, and honey mustard. She nibbled on it throughout the week when she got the munchies.

- A salad or leftover veggies make a great snack. Make extra to nibble on during the week. Try a colorful salad with dressing on the side or broccoli slaw with chopped water chestnuts, red onion, lemon juice, rice vinegar, and 1 tablespoon sesame oil.

 Researchers at the University of Southern California found that if an unhealthy snack is prepared for us, we're more likely to take it. If we have to dish it out ourselves, we're more likely to pass.[6]

Getting in the habit of preparing and eating healthy snacks on a schedule is a game changer when it comes to weight loss. You'll stay full and energized, stay on the Plan, never feel deprived, and keep moving toward your weight-loss goal.

Wedge of Wisdom

When Jamie, one of my middle school clients, gets home from school, she is hungry and ready for a snack. To save calories, she used to skip the bread and eat a scoop of peanut butter. The peanut butter alone didn't satisfy her, so she kept scooping and scooping. When I suggested she schmear 1 tablespoon of peanut butter on a rice cake, whole-grain crackers, or a slice of bread, she noticed a big difference. With her snack portion contained, Jamie felt satisfied and didn't feel the need to eat everything in sight before dinner. This small change, along with snacking on fruit and vegetables, helped her lose 15 pounds.

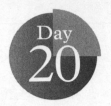

Sip Your Way to Slim

I come from a family where gravy is considered a beverage.
—Erma Bombeck

Sugar-sweetened beverages are the largest source of added sugar and calories in the American diet.[1] And it's no surprise. Sugary drinks are available in large quantities everywhere. Regular soda, fruit drinks, juice cocktails, lemonade, sweetened iced teas, sports drinks, energy drinks, and sweetened waters (including vitamin-enhanced waters!), as well as the many sweetened coffee drinks on the market, all have sugar. And now more than ever there are many healthy-sounding sugary drinks to choose from, including smoothies and protein drinks sweetened with some form of sugar, whether honey, coconut sugar, or maple syrup. We're drinking our calories. And because we swallow rather than chew our beverages, many of us dismiss these calories, treating them almost as if they were freebies.

If you want to lose weight, you've got to look at the liquid in your diet. Most beverages have calories—and some can even have a day's worth. Even a healthy-sounding smoothie can top the 1,000-calorie mark. I'm not suggesting you give up all your favorite beverages. I do have strategies to help some of you cut hundreds of calories out of your day by making small changes to what's going down the hatch.

The simple act of chewing thoroughly helps us feel full. Chewing also aids digestion. We absorb more nutrients, and we give ourselves a chance to decide whether we're full. Researchers at Kyushu University in Japan found that chewing slowly and thoroughly can help us lose weight and prevent obesity.[2] When we drink our calories, the brain doesn't get the same messages it does when we eat. We don't feel as full and we tend to eat more at our next meal.[3] In a Purdue University study, researchers found that fruit juice drinkers, when compared to participants who ate whole fruit, were not as satisfied and ingested more calories throughout the day.[4]

Chew This Over

A tall glass of calories

A good part of the reason people overconsume sugary drinks is the size they come in. A small soda at the movie theater, for instance, can contain more than a quart of liquid. My research tracking the history of soda sizes at fast-food restaurants found that a small soda is more than double the size it was when first introduced. The large sizes can be upward of a quart and even close to ½ gallon. Portion sizes of soft drinks have increased more than the sizes of most other foods, making it far too easy to guzzle down hundreds of calories.[5] Some companies have reduced soda sizes in recent years (7-Eleven downsized its Double Gulp from 64 ounces with nearly 800 calories to 50 ounces with nearly 600 calories, for instance), yet we've still got a long way to go.

Coffee drinks are oversized as well. A 16-ounce grande, or medium, white chocolate mocha Frappuccino at Starbucks clocks in at 440 calories, and even a 12-ounce tall (small) size contains 320 calories! And while nutritionists generally recommend consuming no more than 4 ounces—½ cup—of fruit juice at a time, most people routinely drink at least twice that, and bottled juices are usually sold in 12- or 16-ounce containers.

A Cup of Coffee or a Cup of Calories?

2 ounces of:	Calories
Cream	120
Half-and-half	74
Chocolate milk (whole milk)	52
Whole milk	38
2 percent milk	30
1 percent milk	26
Fat-free milk	22
Soy milk, unsweetened	20
Almond milk, unsweetened	15

Source: USDA

Bite-Sized Goodie A typical 12-ounce can of regular cola contains nearly 10 teaspoons of added sugar; a 20-ounce bottle contains 16 teaspoons of added sugar. One sugary drink a day and you are at or over the recommended level of added sugars.

Sugary beverages, weight gain, and health

There's good reason to cut back on sugary beverages. They have been strongly linked to weight gain and obesity, especially in children.[6] In response to claims that restaurants are contributing to childhood obesity, some restaurants have replaced sugary beverages with bottled water and low-fat milk on children's menus. The availability of sugary drinks on menus decreased by nearly 20 percent between 2008 and 2016.[7] But many restaurants still offer free refills on soda. Most people wouldn't buy a second soda but will gladly take a free refill.

Likewise, cutting back on drinks with added sugar is proven to help you lose weight.[8] A study at Virginia Tech suggests that swapping just one sugary drink per day for water has a huge health benefit. Replacing one sugary drink per day, including "diet" beverages, with water can reduce the risk of obesity and other health conditions.[9]

Sugary drinks also contribute to other health problems. Harvard University researchers learned that eating whole fruits such as blueberries, grapes, and apples may lower the risk of type 2 diabetes, while drinking fruit juice is associated with raising the risk.[10] Researchers from Stellenbosch University in South Africa reported that sugary drinks such as soda and juice can lead to the development of diabetes, high blood pressure, and more.[11]

Skip the diet soda. The research on diet sodas is mixed with regard to weight gain.[12] Some research found that diet drinks are associated with modest increases in weight and waist circumference, while others reported that diet drinks are associated with less weight gain than regular soda. It's important to note that the studies exploring the relationship between diet soda and weight gain are observational studies (and are observing an association between diet soda and weight gain). They don't prove that diet soda, per se, is causing the weight gain. Regardless, drinking diet sodas probably doesn't help you lose weight, and they provide no nutritional value, so opt for water or sparkling water instead.

Take small, slow sips. Researchers at Wageningen University in the Netherlands suggested that small sips lead to better satiety because people believe they are consuming more![13]

THE MANY NAMES OF SUGAR

Read the label and limit these sweeteners:

Agave syrup	Evaporated cane sugar	Honey
Brown rice syrup		Malt syrup
Brown sugar	Fructose	Maltose
Cane sugar	Fruit juice concentrates	Maple syrup
Coconut sugar		Molasses
Corn sweetener	Glucose	Raw sugar
Corn syrup	High-fructose corn syrup	Sucrose
Dextrose		

Make your mouth water

You may feel you need your morning Frappuccino, but when it comes to beverages, your body really only needs water. Water does more than quench your thirst. It keeps your body energized and may even help you lose weight! Virginia Tech researchers found that adults who drank 500 milliliters of water (a little more than 2 cups) before a low-calorie meal over a twelve-week period lost 44 percent more weight than adults who didn't drink as much water.[14] When you drink water, you're also less likely to drink sugary beverages,[15] further contributing to weight loss.

Staying hydrated can prevent constipation, give you healthy-looking skin, and energize muscles. It is even important for brain health. Try to drink somewhere in the ballpark of 64 ounces a day and whenever you're thirsty. If you want some extra flavor, squeeze in some fresh lemon or lime. You can also infuse your water with fruits, vegetables, or herbs. I love a cup of hot water with lemon or cold water infused with berries, cucumbers, or mint leaves. It's natural, soothing, and hydrating. Flavored seltzer water and unsweetened herbal iced teas are also good choices.

Smart Sips: Save 600+ Calories Effortlessly

Drink This	Calories	Instead of This	Calories	Calorie Savings
Tall nonfat latte	100	Venti whole-milk latte	300	200
Orange juice, 4 ounces	58	Orange juice, 16 ounces (1 pint)	234	176
Water	0	Soda, 20 ounces	260	260

Source: USDA

Slice of Advice

Drink water before you go for the juice. Researchers from the University of Hohenheim in Germany found that participants drank 19 percent more water when they poured it first and 25 percent more juice when they poured it first.[16]

Plan-style smoothies

I'm not suggesting you live on water alone. Many beverages without added sugars are filling and healthy. You just have to be aware of what's in your glass. When making a smoothie at home, for instance, use the smallest blender cup available as a way to portion control it. Use whole fruit (up to 1 cup), fresh vegetables, ice for fluff, and either milk, unsweetened yogurt, an unsweetened milk swap, or water. (Greek yogurt, bananas, and ice are great thickeners.) Add vanilla, peanut powder, cinnamon, or almond extract for flavor. Avoid smoothies with avocado, peanut butter, and 100 percent juice, which add extra calories. Skip the fruit punch too. The idea is to keep added sugar out and save fats for cooking and eating.

SODA SUBSTITUTES

Drink sparkling water, seltzer, or club soda with no added sodium instead of soda.

Fill ice cube trays with juice or blended fruit ingredients. Add a few ice cubes to your water or sparkling water.

When ordering a smoothie from a shop, consider the following:

- Order the small.
- Skip the added sugar and fruit juice.
- Check the calorie count on the menu.
- Add greens, which are low in calories and high in nutrients—spinach, kale, cucumbers, and celery.
- Ask for lots of crushed ice.

Bite-Sized Goodie The trick to making a satisfying low-cal smoothie is to make it thick. Researchers from Wageningen University in the Netherlands found that participants who drank a frothy 100-calorie milk shake were fuller than those who drank a thinner shake with 500 calories.[17]

Small changes can make a big difference on the scale. I know many people who've lost 10 or more pounds simply by substituting one sugary drink a day for a healthier option. Rethink what you drink and you, too, can sip your way to slim.

Wedge of Wisdom

Sam was a big soda drinker. He started his day with a Mountain Dew and drank about six cans a day. By the time I met him, he was almost 100 pounds overweight and jittery from all the caffeine and sugar. To lose weight and feel better, he needed to cut out the soda. We started by replacing his last soda of the day with flavored seltzer water, which he enjoyed. He missed his soda but slept better and woke up feeling better. After a couple of weeks, we replaced another soda with seltzer and then two weeks later another. He kept his refrigerator stocked with all types of flavors. He was so happy with how he felt that he endured the initial withdrawal well. Before he realized it, he'd lost about 50 pounds and felt calm and relaxed for the first time in years.

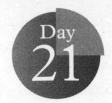

Embrace the 80/20 Rule

All you need is love. But a little chocolate now and then
doesn't hurt.

—Charles M. Schulz

I would guess that a disciplined Olympic-gold-medal-winning diver
sometimes needs to do a cannonball, just for the fun of it. The same
applies to eating and exercise. Every now and then, you just need
to cut loose from your routine and miss a workout, enjoy a bigger
portion, indulge in a food you normally shy away from, or eat out
at your favorite restaurant when you would normally cook at home.
Most people break if they feel sentenced to a lifetime of following
a strict regimen. This may explain why so many people stop dieting after a month or two. So I like to apply the 80/20 rule: Stick to
your plan of eating healthy food and exercising at least 80 percent
of the time, and depart from the usual up to 20 percent of the time.
For many people, having this wiggle room is the most balanced
approach to a healthy diet.

The 80/20 principle is a lifestyle that helps you sustain weight
loss. It is not an exact science but rather teaches balance and moderation in all things. It boils down to having a healthy relationship

with food and exercise—and your long-term goals. When you practice the 80/20 rule, you have the space to go out and enjoy your favorite Italian meal every now and then, a cocktail (yes, an apple martini!), or your favorite party treat and not feel guilty or deprived. You can miss a workout on the occasion when you really, really just feel like cozying up with a book or watching a movie. Psychologically, you set yourself up to stick to a healthy eating plan and exercise program for the long run because you don't have to be perfect. The pressure, in other words, is off.

The forbidden fruit

The 80/20 rule is rooted in research. Telling yourself you can't have something is a sure way to get your mind to focus on wanting it. Conversely, gently allowing yourself a treat keeps you in tune with your body's hunger signals.

Penn State researchers, for instance, found that girls who were allowed small treats every day ate them only if hungry. They were less covetous of treats and tended to weigh less than girls who were not allowed to have treats.[1] Researchers at Maastricht University in the Netherlands also found that restricting fruit and sweet treats only made them more desirable. And tipping toward the other end of the scale is not any better. Children who were allowed to eat as many sweets as they wanted lost touch with their bodies' hunger signals and continued to eat even when full.[2]

Catholic University of Portugal research added yet another dimension to the 80/20 rule. They found that people who *planned* a break from the "extended inhibition of desires" needed for weight loss fared better than those who did not. Dieters who planned their cheats had, overall, more self-control and more motivation and enjoyed the process more than those who didn't plan their cheats.[3]

If you are in the mood for your favorite fun food, consider the delay tactic: Promise yourself you can have the treat in 20 minutes and then see if you still want it. Delay rather than deprive and your craving might just subside.[4]

Track your indulgences in your Portion Tracker— maybe even highlight them. If you see it on paper, you'll notice if you're suddenly following the 50/50 rule.

When it's good to be bad

Do allow yourself to indulge in something small such as a treat up to four times per week, if you feel the need to. And feel free to enjoy two fun meals, such as lasagna or steak, each week if you have the urge.

Do plan your indulgence, or legalize it, which as you know by now is a great way to bar guilt from entering the picture. You keep a balanced mind-set without compromising your weight-loss goals.

Do continue to plan your healthy meals about 80 percent of the time. When you focus on a healthy lifestyle, weight loss is the healthy by-product.

Do make it worth your while. I have found from years of counseling people trying to lose weight that most do best when they plan to have a treat they enjoy after dinner. This treat gives you something to look forward to and helps you to not feel deprived.

Do be kind to yourself and savor the treats or indulgences you plan for. If the urge passes, it's okay to break your plans.

Don't schedule cheat days, or save up treats and have them all on the same day. Not drinking all week and then having seven cocktails over the weekend is good for neither your body nor your healthy relationship with food.

If you apply the 80/20 rule and are not losing weight, try a 90/10 plan. After you lose some weight, you can try the 80/20 rule again.

Food is part of life, and life should be fun at times. The more you enjoy your food plan, the more likely you are to stay on it. So give yourself a scheduled break. You've already earned your gold medal for all the effort you've put into the Finally Full, Finally Slim Program. Reward yourself when the portion is right.

Wedge of Wisdom

Sharon, a thirty-five-year-old stay-at-home mom, had lost and regained weight several times. Sharon followed the all-or-nothing rule. She either diligently followed a diet or succumbed to sugar cravings and started overeating. When she came to see me, we legalized a fun food. She could have either an extra treat or a favorite portion-friendly meal several days of the week. She planned for it and legalized it. When Sharon approached her weight loss as a lifestyle rather than a strict diet she was on or off, her struggles ended. The 80/20 rule was tailor-made for Sharon.

Master Special Occasions

> The secret to living well and longer—eat half, walk double, laugh triple, and love without measure.
>
> —Tibetan proverb

Most people look forward to life's special occasions: weddings, showers, graduations, birthdays, anniversaries, holidays, vacations, picnics, and parties. These events can strike fear into those of us trying to lose weight. Don't let fear of weight gain prohibit you from being the belle of the ball. Whether you're going on a once-in-a-lifetime trip or to a simple gathering, you can enjoy life's celebrations *and* maintain your weight by thinking ahead and mastering a few tips.

The life of the party

A little preparation and strategy can get you through parties and holidays without gaining an ounce.

Expect the best; prepare for the worst.
- Get enough sleep the night before. If you're tired, you might crave sugary foods or eat just to stay awake.

- Decide ahead of time what you will and won't eat or drink. Is this a cheat meal or are you sticking to healthy foods? Will you drink alcohol or sparkling water instead?
- Just as you would when dining out, eat something healthy before you head out so you're not famished and forced to eat something you'd rather not.
- For a potluck, bring a healthy dish to share. If everyone else brings cheesecake and chocolate brownies, you can turn to your kale salad with apples and almonds (if there's any left!).
- If you're the host, treat your guests to a healthy meal. If necessary, make one decadent dish that you know others will expect.
- If you're the host and you don't want the leftovers around, have enough baggies or containers on hand so you can give the food to your guests when they leave.
- For a day or so before and after a big event, eat light and add 10 or 15 minutes more to your exercise routine.
- Get centered before an event. Anticipate who or what might sabotage your efforts to eat healthy. Prepare yourself for an evening of mindful eating.

Be strategic.
- Make people, not food, center stage. Socializing is the main event.
- Be selective. Take a lap around a buffet, just as you would at a buffet in a restaurant.
- Drink lots of water and nurse only one alcoholic beverage.
- Before grabbing a second plate of food, talk to someone new. And drink a glass of water. You may be thirsty, but it is unlikely you are still hungry.
- Wait at least 20 minutes before heading back to the buffet for more food. There's a good chance you will no longer want seconds.
- Go for the berries or other fruit for dessert.

- Exercise in the morning to make sure you get your workout in before the party.
- Dance! You'll burn off calories in no time and have fun doing it.
- Be mindful of how much you're eating in nibbles. Broken cookies and crackers do, indeed, have calories.
- To avoid nibbling, pass by the wandering trays of appetizers. Instead, take a small plate of appetizers and sit down to eat. Calories still count when you eat standing!
- Strike up conversations away from the food spread.

WEIGHT-LOSS-FRIENDLY PARTY FOODS AND DRINKS

Turn to these common party foods if available. They are satisfying and will hold you over. Fruits and veggies are filling and packed with fiber. Chickpeas and edamame contain protein and fiber—the perfect fill-me-up combo. I have also found that tomato juice cuts appetite (and it's low in calories), so it makes for the best cocktail.

Baked sweet potato fries

Bloody Mary

Bruschetta

Chicken kebabs

Crudités and white bean dip

Dry-roasted chickpeas

Edamame

Fruit kebabs

Grilled vegetables

Guacamole with carrots and cucumbers

Hummus and whole-grain pita

Kale chips

Mixed berries

Mixed nuts

Smoked salmon with cherry tomatoes and whole-grain crackers

Sparkling water with lime

Sushi

Tomato juice

Virgin Mary

White wine spritzer

- Celebrations are about more than food and drink. Focus on what you're celebrating.
- Split dessert with someone and enjoy the company.

Bite-Sized Goodie

Despite all the noise people make about holiday weight gain, researchers at the University of Sonora in Mexico found that most adults gain about 1–2 pounds.[1] The holidays are not a time to start a diet. It's more important to get back on track after the holidays.

How much is too much?

The *Dietary Guidelines* suggest that, if you're going to drink alcohol, you do so in moderation.[2] *Moderation* is defined as one drink daily for women and two for men. If you're trying to lose weight, I suggest you limit alcohol to no more than once or twice a week and have it with a meal. (If you don't drink, you can use your treat servings for something else!)

SERVING SIZES FOR ALCOHOL

Wine, 5 ounces

Beer (regular and light), 12 ounces

Distilled spirits (vodka, rum, gin, whiskey, tequila), 1½ ounces

  (Even mixers have calories, so skip the soda and remember to keep track of your mixer.)

Liqueur, 1½ ounces

Vacations, business travel, and road trips

Whether you are going on a road trip or traveling by plane, you can enjoy yourself without departing too much from the Plan. Here's how.

Pack healthy snacks. Plan to pack snacks just like you plan to pack your clothes. (See Day #19: Power Up Your Snacks, page 175, for more ideas.) Choose a combo of fiber (fruits, veggies, whole-grain crackers, rice cakes) and protein (hummus, bean dip, chickpeas, edamame, yogurt, cheese, turkey, egg) or healthy fat (nuts, nut butters, avocado) for maximum fullness. I love taking mini-cans of low-sodium V8 juice—they can go anywhere except in the luggage you carry on board an airplane.

Plan your meals. You'll likely be eating out more often on a trip than you do at home. In many ways, this tactic is no different than planning your meals when you're in your hometown. Going out to a special dinner and want to order your favorite lasagna dish? Work your other meals around it. Have a salad topped with grilled fish, chicken, or your favorite beans for lunch, sans bread. Have some fun with it and make it your mission to try healthy local foods or find healthy restaurants. Enjoy a fun meal and treat on occasion, but choose wisely.

Balance it out. If you overeat today, tighten your portion belt tomorrow.

Stay hydrated. Water, water, water! Herbal tea works too. Flying, especially, can dehydrate you. If you go to a warmer or dryer climate or a higher altitude than you're used to, you may need much more water during your travels. Listen to your body and avoid dehydrating beverages, including coffee and alcohol.

Keep moving! Go into your trip intending to exercise, and pack your workout attire. Have some idea of how you'll stay active. Walk or ride a bike to tourist sites. Attend the early morning spinning class on the cruise ship and walk or run the deck. Take a yoga class at a local

Transportation Security Administration regulations limit what you can bring on an airplane, so think ahead.

Be Airport Smart

Liquids and more. Buy liquids (water, V8), Greek yogurt, single-serve hummus (yes, I've had my hummus confiscated!), and guacamole after you go through the security checkpoint. Or bring an empty water bottle with you and fill it up at a water fountain once you're through security. You can also buy a salad with dressing on the side.

Edibles. Bring part-skim cheese and whole-grain crackers, apples, pears, a container of berries, snack packs of your favorite unsalted nuts, single-serve nut butters, individual oatmeal packs, salmon or tuna in a pouch, and cut-up vegetables for the plane ride. I also never leave home without my favorite herbal tea bags (chamomile and peppermint). Avoid dried meat and jerkies (which are heavily processed and full of sodium) and dried fruit (which is high in sugar and easy to overeat).

Check out Appendix B (page 259), where I provide a longer list of fun and healthy snacks.

studio. Use the hotel swimming pool and workout facility. Go for long walks or plan an early morning run on the beach. Take advantage of local sports—take a scuba or surfing lesson or learn how to ski or snow-shoe. You might discover a new favorite activity. When in Rome...

Request a room with a fridge. Stop at the grocery store just before or shortly after you arrive at your hotel so you can get some healthy foods. You'll save money and calories and won't be at the mercy of the minibar.

Continue to keep your Portion Tracker. It works at any latitude and longitude.

Show it off. If you've lost some weight already, celebrate by wearing some new clothes that fit your new body. Don't even bring your fat clothes. Men, that goes for you, too. Get a new belt or swimsuit.

Get right back on track when you get home. Don't weigh yourself right after a vacation. Give yourself at least a day or two to eat well and exercise.

When you're out of your typical environment, structure is going to go by the wayside. There's no getting around it. Resign yourself to the fact that you may not continue to lose weight during your vacation and that you're going to splurge or that you might over-eat at a party. Researchers at Utrecht University in the Netherlands found that dieters who obsess over indulging ate more junk food than those who cut themselves some slack.[3] Accept your splurge for what it was—fun and delicious. Think maintenance instead. And if you do gain a few pounds, you know how to lose them again. Focus on the goal, stay positive, *enjoy yourself*, and when you get home, get back on track.

Wedge of Wisdom

Mark, a forty-five-year-old real estate developer, travels extensively for work. He practically lives in the airport, which was impeding his weight-loss efforts. Every time he traveled, he'd regain any weight he had lost. At one of our first sessions, we made some plans. He prepared single servings of healthy snacks, including nuts, oatmeal, fruits, and veggies. We identified new go-to foods that he could pur-chase at the airport. We focused on weight maintenance while he traveled. The results? He didn't gain weight while traveling. When he got home, he could start where he left off on the scale.

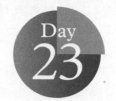

Stay on Track

Believe you can and you're halfway there.

— Theodore Roosevelt

Just when your clothes start to feel a little looser and you're in a rhythm—exercising, preparing healthy foods, and being mindful of everything you've learned in this book so far—it happens. You sprain your ankle while jogging and comfort yourself with a huge slice of chocolate cake, which sets off sugar cravings. Not to mention that jogging, your exercise of choice, is now off-limits for six weeks. Before you know it, you've regained the weight you lost. You mentally beat yourself up for putting in your best effort and tasting success only to land right back where you started. Then you ask yourself, *What's the point of trying to lose weight if it's so easy to regain?*

Regaining weight can have you going from sixty to zero in a New York minute. Yet life is full of events we can't control. When life throws you lemons, make the proverbial lemonade. You are human. You may overeat or get off track. You might think negative thoughts. More important than what happens to you is how you deal with it. The right response can help you to stick to your goals. You ate because you ate. You had a slip. Rather than sink into old habits and head into a full-blown relapse, enjoy your big slice of chocolate cake and then get back on track.

Slip Sliding Away

What's the difference between a slip and a relapse? A slip is buying a family-size bag of chips and eating it in two sittings. You know it's your trigger food. But, upset over a work issue, you couldn't seem to control yourself. You wake up the next morning, acknowledge that the chips didn't serve your weight-loss goals, and decide to exercise a little longer and eat a little less that day. By the following day, you're back on track.

A relapse starts before a slip. You start thinking that all this weight-loss stuff is too much work. You miss one workout one week, then three, and then decide you don't have time to work out and who are you to think you can get into shape. With a relapse, you might spend weeks talking yourself out of your goals, slip, and then give up.

Celebrate your slip. Researchers at the University of Canterbury in New Zealand found that women who felt guilty after eating a big slice of chocolate cake gained more weight than those who felt good after eating it. Women who associated the cake with celebration were more successful in their weight-loss efforts.[1]

It's never too late

Whether you've slipped or gone into a full-blown relapse, be kind to yourself. If you learn from it, you haven't failed. Instead you're one step closer to getting it right. Getting off track tells you that something in your plan needs fixing. Ask yourself what happened. Why did you do it? Did you plan for it? Did you skip a meal? Were your friends eating? Did you even like the food you ate? If you know the why, you can come up with a new how, or a better, more thoughtful response than the one you turned to.

Following are common reasons for derailing and ideas for what you can do instead of slipping:

If you eat for comfort. Pamper yourself with a spa treatment; take a long, luxurious bubble bath; call a dear friend and go for a long walk.

If you eat when stressed. Light a candle and sip some hot chamomile tea; take a yoga or meditation class; write about why you're stressed in a journal.

If you eat when bored. Meet a friend for dinner, complete chores you've been putting off (vacuum, pay bills), move to another room, or go outdoors.

If you eat just because the food is there. Consider whether you need to pay more attention to your Portion Tracker or work on how you can better plan your meals and snacks; revisit Day #9: Declutter Your Kitchen (page 105) and follow the guidelines for how to keep unhealthy foods out of sight and healthy foods front and center.

If you're more hungry than usual. Take advantage of the 80/20 rule.

If you eat because you're tired. Take a short nap or meditate for 5 minutes.

If you eat because you're unmotivated. Play your favorite music.

If you eat out of habit. Create a new habit and begin to practice it (for ideas, see Day #16: Be Your Own General, page 155).

If you eat because everyone else is eating. Stop, and ask yourself, *Am I hungry?* Get in touch with your internal feelings of hunger and don't eat just because the food is available. Or, when possible, choose something healthy. If you are eating because it is a special occasion, enjoy it, and count it as your treat for the day.

If you eat when you're angry. Visualize three things you are grateful for. And visualize yourself at your ideal weight.

If you stop exercising because of time constraints or inter-ferences. Come up with a new exercise schedule or build it into your day by biking to work, for instance.

Direct some compassion toward yourself. Researchers at the University of Portsmouth in the UK found that people who showed self-compassion were more likely to maintain weight loss.[2]

Get out of your own way

I think people who are able to lose weight and keep it off make a leap of faith. They believe they can do it, and they believe they deserve it. If somewhere deep in the recesses of your subconscious mind you have doubts, you might sabotage your weight-loss efforts without even knowing it. Self-sabotage is more common than you might think. Here are some foolproof ways to fight self-sabotage, just in case you've an iota of disbelief:

Set reasonable goals. When we're motivated to lose weight, some of us get all zealous and go overboard with goals. We convince ourselves we can exercise 2 hours a day, six days a week, and lose 20 pounds in two weeks. With all-or-nothing approaches, we usually end up with nothing. We set ourselves up for failure. Instead, start out small and grow into your changes. If you now exercise three days a week, exercise for four. If you now drink two glasses of wine when dining out, try replacing one with sparkling water. It's okay to approach weight loss at a pace you know you can manage. Inching your way toward your goal is better than setting yourself up to fail.

Keep the promises you make to yourself. Nothing says dis-belief like a trail of broken promises. If you say you're going to do something, do it. Set negative thoughts and fears aside and focus on the promise. Keeping your word to yourself, even when you're unsure of yourself, is a show of self-respect and confidence. Put your workout on the calendar and forget about your excuses. Most excuses are fear in disguise. Do what you say you will do, and before you know it, you'll have new, healthy, and enjoyable habits.

Be yourself. I love this quote from Nelson Mandela: "There is no passion to be found in playing small—in settling for a life that is less than the one you are capable of living." If we're used to living in the shadow of others, or if our friends are not as supportive as we'd like, we can sabotage even the most important of personal goals to avoid success. It's possible to intentionally fail because we don't want to appear better than those around us. Your losing weight has nothing to do with anyone but you. This is your goal, your health, and your life.

 Stanford University School of Medicine researchers learned that women who had the support of family and friends were 26 percent more likely to lose weight than women who didn't have support.[3]

The secret to maintaining weight loss

It's no secret that many people regain the weight they lose on a diet. They start out motivated, they are applauded by family and friends, and once they reach their goal and their focus shifts, their weight creeps back up. I see many people who approach weight loss with this well-known fact in mind. Weight regain is a reality for many people. Researchers at the Warren Alpert Medical School of Brown University recorded results of seventy overweight or obese adults who completed a twelve-week weight-management program. Each participant lost about 1 pound a week. Almost immediately after ending the program, participants starting regaining about .15 pound per week.[4]

Healthy behaviors and habits can help to set you apart. Weight loss and maintenance are as much about food as they are about behavior. Researchers tracking what makes "losers" successful in the National Weight Control Registry found that continued adherence to diet and exercise strategies as well as maintaining the behavior changes they made when losing weight were associated with long-term success.[5] Some healthy practices of these "losers" were: exercising regularly, maintaining a consistent eating pattern on weekdays and weekends, weighing themselves at least once a week, eating breakfast, and following a low-calorie, low-fat diet.[6]

Portion control, healthy food choices, exercise, planning, and eating mindfully are just a few of the new behaviors you've learned in this book so far. If you slip or relapse, go back to them. Reread this book. Revisit your Portion Tracker. Remember why you wanted to lose weight in the first place. Maintaining weight loss is *absolutely possible* when your mind-set, environment, and habits—your life— are in unison with healthy food choices and portions. Keep this in mind if you slip or regain. You know what to do.

Wedge of Wisdom

Annie, my client and an ex-splurger, bought me a poster with this saying: "A splurge of 1,000 calories begins with a single nibble." Your nibble doesn't have to turn into 1,000 calories. Accept it and move on. Annie would go on and off a diet with a single splurge. She had an on-or-off mentality with her weight-loss plan. After I told her she did not have to be perfect 100 percent of the time, she was able to continue to lose weight even after the occasional ice cream cone.

STAGE 4
Your Life

DAY **24** Step It Up

DAY **25** Sleep Deep

DAY **26** Unplug to Unwind

DAY **27** Love and Connect

DAY **28** Stretch Your Horizons

DAY **29** Pursue Your Passion

DAY **30** Start Each Day Anew

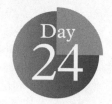

Step It Up

Happiness is a state of activity.
—Aristotle

Most experts agree that it is best to eat a healthy diet and exercise regularly to lose weight. I look at exercise as a game changer, the factor that gets you to the weight-loss and maintenance tipping point. Researchers at the University of the State of Rio de Janeiro found that when combined with a healthy food plan, increased physical activity leads to a 20 percent greater weight loss than diet *or* exercise alone. Study participants who employed both methods also sustained their weight loss for at least one year.[1]

Exercise has positive effects all around. In addition to helping with weight loss, it improves brain health, joints, and sleep. Exercising reduces stress and the risk for chronic diseases, including heart disease, certain cancers, diabetes, high blood pressure, and osteoporosis. It helps stabilize blood sugar as well as improve cholesterol levels. Engaging in regular physical activity also improves mood, which may lead you to make better food choices. It can also reduce appetite. In short, exercise makes you fit. You feel happy, healthy, strong, and confident. The key is to make it fun and keep doing it.[2]

 Consider joining a health club or signing up for a series of classes, whether it be cycling, yoga, or Zumba. University of Pennsylvania researchers found that attending an exercise class can foster a little competition and motivate participants to exercise.[3]

What is fitness?

When you're fit, you feel healthy and strong. You can achieve this by combining different types of exercises to strengthen your heart, lungs, and muscles; improve bone density and metabolism; and much, much more.

Following are four components of fitness:

1. Cardio (aerobic/endurance): swimming, vinyasa yoga, jogging, brisk walking, biking, hiking, dancing, spinning, Zumba
2. Strength training: weight lifting, body conditioning, certain types of yoga, barre classes
3. Flexibility: yoga, Pilates, stretching
4. Balance: yoga, Pilates, barre classes

Want to enjoy your workout even more? Listen to music. Researchers at Brunel University London in the UK found that listening to upbeat music while exercising led to a 28 percent increased enjoyment in exercise when compared to the enjoyment level of exercisers who didn't listen to music.[4]

How much exercise do you need?

To enjoy the benefits of exercise, you don't need to run a marathon. You just need to move your body. Guidelines call for 150 minutes (2½ hours) of moderate-intensity aerobic activity (brisk walking, swimming), 75 minutes of vigorous-intensity aerobic activity (jogging, tennis), or an equivalent mix of the two each week, plus strength train-ing twice a week.[5] But it all depends on your current level of fitness.

Goodie Want stronger bones in 60 seconds? Researchers from the University of Exeter in the UK found that short bursts of exercise—such as jogging up the stairs or doing jumping jacks—throughout the day help protect bone health.[6]

Your ultimate goal is to exercise most days of the week. Aim for *at least* four to five days a week, 30–45 minutes at a time. You can do more, too. It depends on your schedule and current activity level. If you already have a regular exercise program, keep it up and change it up. Trying different exercises may even help crank up your metabolism. If you're pretty much sedentary, start small and work your way up to the recommendation. Diving into a new exercise plan head on can backfire. If you do too much too soon, you might feel tired or sore and give up. So start slow. No matter what your current activity level, you can do something. Walk the dog for a couple of blocks, do simple arm and leg stretches at your desk, park your car at the far end of the grocery store lot, get off the bus or sub-way several stops before your destination, or walk to the restaurant and back. After a week, increase your walk by a couple of blocks or tackle the hill that's just down the road.

Almost any activity can burn calories—and add up through-out the day. Researchers at Rovira i Virgili University in Spain found that overweight older adults (ages fifty-five to seventy-five) reduced obesity and were most fit when they exercised regularly but also when they kept their heart rate up throughout the day with "moderate-vigorous" activity.[7] So keep moving.

Research results vary regarding how much and what type of exercise we need in order to lose weight or maintain weight loss and improve health. My advice? Do what you love. You're more likely to stick with it.

Slice of Advice Walking is great exercise. It's free (except for a small investment in a good pair of walking shoes), you don't have to be an athlete, you can join a friend, and it's good for brain health! For an added health boost, speed up your pace.[8]

Bite-Sized Goodie Take ten! University of Nevada researchers found that multiple 10-minute bouts of exercise can have an effect similar to that of one longer workout for improving heart health and endurance. So no excuses! It's easy to find 10 minutes three to four times a day.[9]

Do what you love, regularly

I love to practice yoga, swim, and bike. I get bored, however, on treadmills and other stationary equipment. Because I do what I enjoy, I keep coming back. You'd be hard-pressed to talk me out of going to my yoga class, where I look forward not only to the workout but to socializing with my fellow yogis who show up regularly. Because it's fun to me, I go consistently. And that's important. Drexel University researchers learned that developing a *consistent schedule* of healthy eating and exercise is key to losing weight.[10] (See Day #16: Be Your Own

STRETCH IT OUT

Yoga is known for helping people relax and get centered. Its benefits don't stop there. Yoga improves body awareness and body image and enforces mindfulness. When you leave the mat, you're more likely to stay mindful—and that includes at the dinner table. Research found that people who practice yoga for only 30 minutes per week, for at least four years, gain less weight and may even lose weight.[11]

General, page 155, for more on how to plan for exercise.) Once you're in a routine, don't be afraid to vary it by trying something new. Join a class or a tennis league, find new trails to bike or hike, or schedule an appointment with a personal trainer.

Work out with a buddy. A friend keeps you accountable and makes it more fun. Joining a class can have the same effect and introduces you to new, like-minded people.

Wearable fitness devices

You don't need a Fitbit or other wearable fitness device to lose weight, but you might find them useful. These devices are all the rage and for good reason. They are fun, challenge you to continue moving, and keep you motivated. Use them to mark progress; just don't take all the data literally. Researchers at Hankyong National University in South Korea compared five different devices. While all were within 10 percent accuracy for number of steps taken, the accuracy varied for other factors, including type of exercise (some were poor at tracking stair climbing, for example), calories, and sleep.[12] The same goes for calorie counters on stationary exercise machines, which are likely off as well.

How many steps should you see on your Fitbit or other exercise-tracking device? Fitbit fans will tell you they shoot to see 10,000 steps, or 5 miles, on their trackers every day. Researchers from the University of Warwick in the UK upped the ante to 15,000, or 7–8 miles. The researchers compared the health and waistlines of postal workers in Glasgow who walked from house to house delivering the mail with those who sat at their desks on the job. It was no surprise that those who delivered the mail had smaller waistlines and less risk of heart disease than those who were sedentary. But 15,000 steps was the magic number for zero risk factors for heart disease.[13]

If you want to see a difference on the scale, watch your portions and move your body. The key is to keep your exercise fun and make it a part of your routine. It's that simple.

Wedge of Wisdom

Matt, a thirty-eight-year-old accountant, would head to the gym most evenings after work. His goal was to lose weight and increase muscle mass. He was convinced that protein drinks were key to his success. His upscale gym recommended them (and sold them at the café), so why not? What he didn't realize is that they were slowing his weight loss. He'd guzzle 24 ounces a day, his cup filled with protein powder along with other ingredients, some high in calories—peanut butter, orange juice, and more. We determined that he was getting too many calories from these drinks and could substitute protein-rich foods without the unwanted calories—yogurt with fruit; a fruit smoothie with milk; chicken, turkey, nuts, and eggs. It's better to get your protein from food than to use protein powders. Protein powders are not really necessary if you have access to a healthy diet. If you do have an occasional protein drink, choose whey or pea protein powders over soy-based powders.

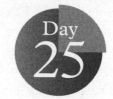

Sleep Deep

Think in the morning. Act in the noon. Eat in the evening.
Sleep in the night.

—William Blake

The connection between diet, exercise, and weight loss is well-known. But researchers have added quality of sleep to the mix as well. Some have found that lack of adequate sleep and being overweight go hand in hand. When we're tired, we're more likely to make poor food choices.[1] Skimping on sleep can even trigger next-day munchies.

Slice of Advice

The National Sleep Foundation recommends that adults get 7–9 hours of sleep. Teenagers do best with 8–10 hours, and school-aged children need 9–11 hours.[2]

A study by researchers at King's College London found that when people got an extra hour of sleep every night, they consumed less sugar compared to people who slept 5–7 hours.[3] When University of Pennsylvania researchers limited study participants to 4 hours of sleep a night for five days, the participants ate more and gained weight.[4] Research on children produced similar results. University of Warwick researchers found that children and adolescents who regularly slept less than others of the same age gained more weight when they grew older and were more likely to become overweight or obese.[5]

Quality sleep leaves us feeling refreshed. We're more positive, better able to concentrate, and more accurately able to follow our food and exercise plans. Sleep even helps the brain work more efficiently so we're ready to learn.[6] Yet, about one-third of Americans don't get enough sleep, and it's affecting their health. According to the Centers for Disease Control and Prevention, poor sleeping habits are linked not only to obesity but to diabetes, heart disease, and depression as well.[7]

During the day

What you do during the day impacts whether you get quality z's at night. Be mindful of the following:

Caffeine. A good cutoff time is noon. Caffeine's stimulating effects can last anywhere from 8 to 14 hours, so the earlier you drink your java, the better.

Alcohol. While a nightcap might make you sleepy, it can reduce the quality of your sleep.

Exercise. Regular exercise promotes sleep. Just avoid doing an intense workout right before bedtime—you might feel energized by it.

Think light. Late-night dinners or snacks should be light and nutritious. Heavy meals and fatty foods are harder to digest. Sugary, salty, and overly spicy foods can also keep you awake.

Be consistent. Try to go to bed and wake up at the same time every day so your body gets used to a schedule. Avoid burning the candle at both ends.

Meditate. It has been shown to improve quality of sleep.

Get outdoors. Going outdoors early in the day promotes better sleep at night.

Can eating certain foods help you sleep?

The research on sleep-promoting foods is inconclusive. While most of us blame the tryptophan (an amino acid thought to induce sleepiness) in turkey for our lethargy after a traditional Thanksgiving dinner, our fatigue may actually result from having eaten too much food. Yet certain foods *do* contain natural substances that may help promote a good night's sleep.[8] Following is a list of foods commonly thought to help you doze off. While we don't know the exact mechanism or extent to which these foods may help you, they are healthy and worth trying if you need help sleeping well.

Warm milk. Just like that nap-inducing Thanksgiving turkey, warm milk contains tryptophan. It also has some melatonin, the sleep hormone that regulates your internal clock. Though tryptophan and melatonin are linked to improved sleep, sleep experts point out that drinking warm milk may have more psychological than physical significance. The routine of drinking a cup of warm milk before bed may bring back childhood memories, which may help us to relax.[9]

Kiwifruit. In one study, subjects who ate two kiwifruits 1 hour before bedtime every night for four weeks fell asleep 35 percent faster than those who didn't eat the New Zealand fruit.[10] The high antioxidant levels (kiwifruit is a good source of vitamins C and E) as well as its B vitamin folate content may explain kiwifruit's sleep-promoting mechanism.[11] Folate deficiency has been linked with insomnia and restless legs syndrome.

Tart cherries. The melatonin, anti-inflammatory properties, and phytonutrient profile of tart cherries have been associated with improved sleep quality.[12] People who drank ¼ cup (4 tablespoons) of tart cherry juice concentrate for seven days slept around 40 minutes longer each night than those who drank a placebo.[13] In a small study, people with insomnia who started drinking tart cherry juice got an additional hour of sleep each night.[14]

Good Night, Moon Milk

The latest rage in natural sleep aids is moon milk, or warm milk spiced with nonalcoholic sleep-inducing agents such as tart cherry juice concentrate or turmeric, black pepper, and cinnamon. Tart cherries contain a natural source of melatonin. Just 1 ounce (2 tablespoons) of tart cherry juice concentrate contains the juice of more than sixty cherries. Turmeric helps to reduce inflammation, and black pepper helps the body absorb turmeric, so the combination can work well. Moon milk hasn't been proven to work as a sleep aid, but if it works for you, go for it—but only if it's worth the extra calories.

Fatty fish. Fish such as salmon and tuna are good sources of omega-3 fatty acids and vitamin D, nutrients that may help regulate serotonin, a neurotransmitter made from the amino acid tryptophan, which helps to regulate sleep, mood, and other functions.[15]

Bananas. Bananas contain the minerals magnesium and potassium, which may work to relax muscles and help promote sleep.

Nuts and seeds. Nuts and seeds contain healthy fats and the muscle-relaxing mineral magnesium. Almonds and walnuts contain melatonin. Pumpkin seeds contain substantial amounts of tryptophan.

Herbal tea. A hot cup of tea is soothing and can help you to unwind and relax. Good nighttime teas include chamomile, lavender, lemon balm, passionflower, valerian, and hop.

Turkey. In addition to containing tryptophan, turkey is rich in protein, which helps to stabilize blood sugar. If your blood sugar drops too low during the night, it can wake you up.

Cheese and crackers. Light snacks made of carb-and-protein combos are good choices before bed. The protein in cheese provides sleep-inducing tryptophan, while the carbs in crackers may help you fall asleep faster. Gram for gram, cheddar cheese contains more tryptophan than turkey!

Hummus. Chickpeas, the main ingredient in hummus, are rich not only in tryptophan but also in folate and vitamin B6. Folate helps to regulate sleep patterns, especially in older people, and vitamin B6 helps to regulate your body clock.

Bite-Sized Goodie

If you're going to read immediately before bedtime, read a printed book rather than an e-book. Researchers at Brigham and Women's Hospital found that the blue light emitted from electronic devices keeps us alert and interferes with the body's natural sleep and wake patterns.[16]

Counting sheep... and more

When you're ready for some shut-eye, counting sheep is the traditional way to take your mind off racing thoughts and pressing matters that might be keeping you awake. If you have trouble falling or staying asleep, here are some more current tips:

Clear your mind. Meditate for 5–10 minutes or write down tomorrow's to-do list as a way to let it go for the night. Before going to bed, avoid people, conversation topics, and things that are likely to induce stress.

Prepare with bedtime rituals. Do something soothing. Drink hot herbal tea or take a hot bath with calming essential oils such as lavender or chamomile to relax your muscles.

Fashion a sleep sanctuary. A clean, clutter-free bedroom, fresh linens, black-out shades, temperatures somewhere in the sixties, and a pink-noise or white-noise machine create a calm, sleep-friendly environment. Move TVs and computers elsewhere. Wearing an old-fashioned sleep mask (eye pads—not to be confused with iPads!) may help if you are sensitive to any light that can get through the cracks.

 To figure out why you don't sleep well, keep a sleep diary. Note the food you eat, the time of your last meal, the time you go to bed, the time you wake up, and how you feel in the morning. Knowing your patterns is useful. You might find that something as simple as going to bed an hour earlier or later might give you a better night's sleep.

Lack of sleep eventually interferes with all aspects of life, including weight loss, so it's important to prioritize your z's. If you have trouble sleeping and have tried everything under the sun (or moon), consider seeing a sleep specialist.

Wedge of Wisdom

Stacey, an overweight mom of three, kept very poor sleep habits. She would nibble at night while watching TV, not be able to fall asleep, and then wake up exhausted. So when she got her kids off to school, she'd eat more, thinking it would give her energy. I asked her to keep a basic sleep diary within her Portion Tracker and we identified a few patterns: irregular sleep habits, excess sugar consumption at night, and periodic nightcaps. With encouragement, Stacey tweaked some habits. Instead of sugary snacks and a glass of wine at night, she tried chamomile tea and kiwifruit. She also made it a priority to go to bed earlier and get at least 7 hours of sleep. After doing this for a few weeks, she felt more energized in the morning and ate healthier as well, which helped speed up her weight loss.

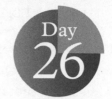

Unplug to Unwind

Your mind will answer most questions if you learn to relax and wait for the answer.

—William Burroughs

In Day #24, I asked you to step it up. Now I want you to step away. It's no secret that chronic stress is rampant in our society. The effects of stress are not always as obvious. Chronic stress taxes us physically and mentally. It can lead to insomnia, high blood pressure, diabetes, depression, anxiety, and even overeating and weight gain.[1]

Much stress comes from the technology meant to make our lives easier. The rapid pace of communication and the expectation to respond to e-mails and texts 24/7, no matter where we are, creates an undercurrent of stress that's hard to escape. Intentionally taking time every day to unplug and unwind reduces stress, puts you in tune with your body, and can make urges to overeat vanish.

Stress and your weight

Stress is known to initially speed up metabolism, but chronic stress can increase how much you eat and ultimately lead to weight gain. People with high levels of stress tend to crave high-calorie, sugary, and fatty foods. They also often have more trouble sleeping, which, as we learned in Day #25: Sleep Deep (page 215), can increase how much you eat and result in weight gain.[2] Ohio State University researchers found that stressed-out women burned fewer calories and had higher insulin levels (which have been linked to obesity) than those who weren't stressed. By the researchers' calculations, chronic stress can slow down metabolism enough to increase the number on the scale by several pounds every year.[3] Regardless of the exact mechanism and relationship between stress, metabolism, and weight, regular stress offers no redeeming qualities, and any measures you take to reduce it are warranted.

Disconnect to reconnect

We all know the many benefits of technology—real-time communication, quick money transfers, and information at our fingertips, to name a few. The downsides? It can disconnect us from the rest of our lives. For some, social media, headline news pings, texts, and e-mail are a constant distraction, interruptive, and overstimulating and steal our attention from tasks and the people around us. When the downsides of technology outweigh the benefits, it's time to disconnect.

You plan your meals and workouts. Now I want you to think about planning daily technology breaks. It's important for your overall well-being, helps you focus on what you're doing (including eating a meal), allows you to be present with the people around you, gives you some control over technology (rather than vice versa), gives you time to think, and puts you in a healthier, happier state of mind. All of this reduces stress. Researchers at the University of British Columbia found that study participants given access to e-mail only three times a day were less stressed than participants given unlimited access to e-mail.[4]

Consider how you can disconnect to reconnect. Here are some suggestions:

Decide what you need to disconnect from. Social media, news, e-mail, texting, anything with a screen?

Schedule routine breaks. Determine when you're usually ready for a break and schedule it. Leave your smartphone behind every time you eat or go to your child's hockey game, for instance. Put your phone and laptop to bed every evening at least 1–2 hours before bedtime. Set aside 30–60 minutes every day to focus on anything other than technology. Do what makes sense for you.

Abstain for a day. Some restaurants have Tech-Free Sundays. They turn off the Wi-Fi so patrons can focus on food, friends, and family. You can do the same at home. Abstain for a full 24 hours or an entire weekend and feel the difference. You might even return to an old tech-free hobby. I don't check e-mail on Saturdays and I am grateful for this much-needed break, especially since I plow through several hundred e-mails in just one day. Perhaps try skipping e-mail for one full day over the weekend. You probably won't miss much other than the latest sale at Bloomingdale's and daily deals from Groupon. E-mail is meant to be a more passive form of communication than a phone call or text. If someone needs your attention now, they'll find another way to contact you.

 Having trouble cutting the cord? There's an app for that. Several apps are available to block access to technology, either on your computer or your cell phone. Check out Cold Turkey, BreakFree, Moment, and others.

Snacks for the soul: The three Ms

I am a huge fan of the three Ms: meditation, music, and massage. They help me unwind, reduce stress, and keep me mindful. If you don't already, try using them to manage stress. Consider them snacks for the soul.

Meditation. I believe in the mind-body connection as it relates to health. Just like you need to be in touch with your hunger, you need to be in touch with your soul. This makes you whole—and reduces stress. Research has shown that meditation, whether sitting in stillness, practicing mindfulness, or doing mindful breathing exercises, may reduce general anxiety, as well as situational stress[5] such as test anxiety.[6] University of Wisconsin researchers found an important physical change: Consistent meditation shrinks the gray matter of the brain associated with stress and conditions the brain to remain calm in the presence of stress.[7] In addition to managing stress, meditation produces immediate benefits. It may make you happy and help you sleep better.

Working meditation into your day is easier than you might think. I try to go to a meditation class about once a week. Meditating with a group of people improves my focus. On most nights, I use a meditation app and get centered for 5–10 minutes. Apps I love are Calm, Omvana, the Mindfulness App, Headspace, and Insight Timer. I'm also naturally drawn to exercises that put me into a bit of a meditative state: Swimming and yoga both get me into the zone.

Bite-Sized Goodie

To meditate, all you need is a quiet place, 5 minutes, and yourself. Sit with good posture, close your eyes or focus on an object about 3 feet away, and then turn your attention to your breathing. Take slow, deep, comfortable breaths. Your mind will wander. When it does, bring it back by focusing on your breathing again. You can do this almost anywhere—in the office, on the subway, while waiting for the dentist, or in the comfort of your home.

Music. I am a huge music nut. It helps me focus. I tend be more productive when listening to music that I enjoy. I even write best while listening to music. The right music for me is calming and even healing. Listening to music before I go to bed relaxes me. The key is to listen to music you enjoy. I love music so much that I spend time making playlists on Spotify. The time I spend is so worth it for my soul and productivity. University of South Alabama researchers found that students who listened to music of their choice or classical music after a stressful test were less anxious than students who listened to heavy metal or nothing at all.[8]

Massage therapy. In addition to relaxing muscles and relieving stress, the ancient practice of massage can help with digestive disorders, as well as headaches, difficulty sleeping, circulation, and joint pain. Even a 10-minute massage is worth your time. Researchers found that mini-massages decrease muscle inflammation after a workout and may even slow the aging process and help prevent obesity. Massage also reinforces the mind-body connection. For relaxation, schedule a massage once or twice a month if you can, or after intense workouts.[9]

MORE SNACKS FOR THE SOUL

Try adding at least one of these stress-reducing activities to your daily routine:

- Stretch.
- Practice being grateful.
- Take a soothing bath.
- Use essential oils—lavender, chamomile, and neroli are calming; lemon and grapefruit are uplifting. Consider purchasing an essential oil diffuser. They add a light scent to your room.
- End your meal with hot herbal tea or hot water with lemon. I love the taste and soothing effects of chamomile and lavender teas.

Research has shown that postmenopausal women who received a weekly 1-hour full-body massage and who massaged their abdomens twice a day with essential oils had lost significant abdominal fat when compared to women who received weekly massages but used grape-seed oil on their abdomens.[10] More research is needed to determine whether essential oils help with weight loss. Pick out an essential oil with a scent you enjoy from a reputable brand and give it a try!

If you're living in a constant state of stress, you're hampering your weight-loss efforts. Unplugging to unwind is essential to achieving peace of mind, which goes hand in hand with weight loss.

Wedge of Wisdom

Natalie came to me wanting to lose 15 pounds. Thirty-nine years old, she longed to be her ideal weight by her fortieth birthday. She would lose weight and then wake up craving food. She couldn't seem to stop nibbling until she gained the weight back. I asked her to try meditating. She at first thought it was silly. "How can I lose weight by sitting?" But she gave it a try. During one particularly meaningful meditation, the answer to her weight-loss struggles just came to her. She realized that her biggest fear was putting in all the effort to lose weight only to gain it back. She expected to fail. Once she understood her mind-set, we came up with ways to turn her subconscious beliefs around. She practiced saying daily affirmations. And, if she felt like sabotaging her progress, she'd remind herself that failure is a thought. It doesn't have to be a reality.

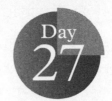

Day
27

Love and Connect

> If I am not for myself, who will be for me? But if I am only
> for myself, who am I?
>
> —Hillel

Brigham Young University researchers followed middle-aged people for seven years to see what factors contributed most to their longevity. The top two most important factors had to do not with physical health but with social life. Having close relationships with people we can depend on is number two. Number one? The short, casual conversations and greetings we have with people we encounter throughout the day—the cashier, the postal worker, the people in our yoga class.[1]

The many benefits to having good friends and connecting with others—even if it's just through a smile—go beyond longevity. Connecting with others in positive ways makes us feel we belong, brightens our day, and generally makes us happier and healthier. Being involved with and helping others matters too.

The right crowd

Whom we hang out with may even impact our weight, weight-loss efforts, and eating habits. When researchers at the University of

Sheffield in the UK reviewed the literature on weight and social networks, they found that friends and family; the community in which we live; the places where we grocery shop and dine out; our peers, including coworkers or students; and our cultural group may all influence weight, physical activity, and how well we eat.[2]

While research has associated the social network phenomenon to the spread of obesity,[3] more recent research extends it to the spread of insulin resistance. The researchers found that lifestyles of social peer groups may influence weight and health.[4] While more research is needed in this area, the idea is that if you spend time with like-minded, health-conscious individuals, you will probably have an easier time sticking to a healthy program than if you hang with couch potatoes.

CAN YOUR DOG HELP YOU LOSE WEIGHT?

I spend lots of time walking my dog—and that's in addition to my regular exercise routine—and it turns out it pays off. Researchers at the Wellness Institute, Northwestern Memorial Hospital in Chicago found that dogs are not only people's best friend but they inspire their owners by being great exercise buddies. According to one study, having a furry companion increases exercise time by at least 3½ hours per week.[5] But that is only if you actually walk your dog! Pet owners also tend to be happier and to be less lonely and stressed and may even live longer than people who do not have pets.[6]

Love yourself first

Many of us are hard on ourselves when it comes to our weight and other aspects of our lives. We might cut ourselves off from social activities for fear of being judged or wear clothes designed to hide love handles rather than make a fashion statement. We're our worst critics. To take advantage of the benefits of connecting with others, self-acceptance is in order. Research found that self-acceptance may also be a precursor to self-improvement. When we accept ourselves, even practices such as mindfulness are more effective than they are for people who tend to be hard on themselves.[7] Self-acceptance gives us greater confidence in our ability to succeed. This may include sticking to our food plan and believing we can do it.

The key to escaping from self-criticism is to accept ourselves, unconditionally, for all that we are. Acceptance is the first step toward change. If we deny that something is, how can we change it?

Self-acceptance goes beyond body image. It's about believing we are capable of doing what we set our minds to. And it's about being able to bear negative criticism without taking it personally. The more we accept ourselves, the easier it is to develop relationships. Nothing in life can serve as a substitute for connecting with others. To increase well-being, we need to care about others and be open to receiving care from others.[8] That includes from ourselves. When we enjoy our own company, others are more likely to enjoy it as well.

I like to think of self-acceptance as self-care. Self-care can mean different things to different people: being mindful, eating healthfully, exercising, not judging ourselves, or making sure we take on only what we can handle. Thinking in terms of self-care centers us. We're more likely to treat ourselves with kindness and respect. To me, self-care also means being involved in your community.

Slice of Advice Laugh your way to good health. University of Maryland researchers found that laughter relaxes blood vessels and promotes a healthy blood pressure.[9] Laughter may also reduce stress, boost your mood, diminish pain, and strengthen your immune system.[10] All without negative side effects!

How we feel about ourselves can change the brain. Researchers from the University of Salzburg in Austria looked at the brains of healthy adults and found that people who accept themselves have more gray matter in the brain region responsible for stress and emotions—and therefore more control over their emotions—than people with low self-esteem.[11]

The power of community

If you feel disconnected from others, try reaching out in your community. Start by doing something positive for others. Volunteer at a soup kitchen, get involved in a local charity, or visit an ill neighbor. Use your talents (we all have them!) to help others. Being active in your community can also protect against loneliness and social isolation, which can adversely affect heath.[12]

My community is an integral part of my life. I volunteer my nutrition services and regularly lecture at my synagogue, where I am also very involved in a women's learning group, among other activities. This and other associations have provided me with many meaningful experiences and friends I can count on. I can't imagine my life without these people and the bonds we've created. Without question, they enrich my life.

As we discussed at the beginning of this chapter, the short encounters we have with members of our community are equally beneficial—the brief chat we have with another dog owner in the park or the smile we show to a passerby. These are what are known as "micro-moments of positive connections." And they're more significant than you probably realize. Connecting in these small ways fights against stress and depression and improves cardiovascular health. Connecting can help us live to a healthy, ripe old age.[13]

Foster some compassion

In *The Art of Happiness*, the Dalai Lama writes, "If you want others to be happy, practice compassion; and if you want yourself to be happy, practice compassion." Self-acceptance comes from self-compassion. So be kind to yourself. Loving ourselves gives us the capacity to love and connect with others. It can even help us lose weight. Researchers at Bishop's University in Canada found that people who practiced self-compassion ate better, exercised more, slept well, and stressed less.[14] Another study from Louisiana State University showed that people who exercised self-compassion after eating a doughnut before a meal ate less when compared to those who weren't asked to exercise self-compassion.[15]

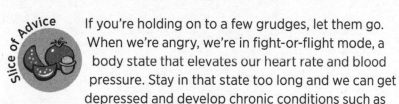 **Slice of Advice** If you're holding on to a few grudges, let them go. When we're angry, we're in fight-or-flight mode, a body state that elevates our heart rate and blood pressure. Stay in that state too long and we can get depressed and develop chronic conditions such as heart disease and diabetes. Find ways to forgive and forget that work for you. It may not always be easy, but it can improve your outlook and well-being.[16]

Good health and how we feel about ourselves are only part of the happiness equation. To lead a full—and long—life, we need to love ourselves and connect with others.

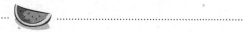

Wedge of Wisdom

My client Debra was an emotional eater. She often ate junk food without realizing it whenever someone wronged her or she felt hurt.

After identifying this pattern, I urged her to work on practicing forgiveness. For Debra, a religious person, praying was the answer. By saying a kind prayer for anyone she felt slighted by, she released her anger. This played a big role for Debra to help stop her emotional eating!

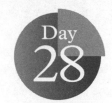

Stretch Your Horizons

To ensure good health: Eat lightly, breathe deeply, live moderately, cultivate cheerfulness, and maintain an interest in life.

—William Londen

One of my favorite fables is the story of two frogs, a well, and an ocean. One day, an ocean frog wanders off and falls into a well, where he meets another frog. The well frog is happy for the company and invites the ocean frog to stay and live with him. Surprised, the ocean frog explains that his home in the ocean is vast and huge and full of exciting adventures. He asks whether the well frog would prefer to come live with him, but the well frog hesitates. He cannot comprehend such a place. He only knows his isolated life in the well. He cannot imagine a world beyond the walls of his well.

This is one of the many versions of the frog story. My point is to encourage you to get out of the well and enjoy something out of your comfort zone, even if you can't imagine what it would be like. When you take a leap (no pun intended) of faith, you risk some discomfort. But stretching your horizons, even just a little, also comes with rewards. Novel experiences stimulate the brain and even enhance learning.[1] And they keep life—and you—interesting.

234 FINALLY FULL, FINALLY SLIM

Trying something new forces you to learn and grow. Every time you challenge yourself, you face fears or obstacles, big and small. These kinds of breakthroughs are inspirational not only to yourself but to others. When you are out of your comfort zone, you learn a little bit about yourself. You may even meet new people, which leads to more new experiences. Growing as a person is exciting and attractive. You are being courageous and proactive. Trying new things results in a feeling of accomplishment—remember this feeling and apply it to all your goals, including weight loss.

Living well doesn't stop when a weight-loss goal is reached. To achieve health, wellness, and a full life, we need to periodically stretch our horizons. The two areas of life I'm going to stress as they relate to your health are that you expand your culinary experiences and your connection to nature.

Get your vitamin N

I love the feeling of being outdoors in nature because it makes me feel at peace and helps me clear my head. I live in New York City and take advantage of our parks, where I take bike rides and long walks. For variety, I take different paths. Some of my most pleasant walks are in Central Park. I also love everything about water— swimming in it and even looking at it. I am lucky to live near the picturesque Carl Schurz Park on the Upper East Side of Manhattan, along the East River. I regularly walk along the promenade, which provides beautiful views of the river. I also relax on the park's plentiful green space with a book, a newspaper, or even some work to read. On those days, I feel restored.

Getting out into the great outdoors has proven to lower stress and reduce symptoms of depression and anxiety. It can leave you feeling restored, even if only in an urban park setting.[2] Researchers at the University of California–San Francisco gave low-income families park maps, bus schedules, and a "prescription" to get out-doors. The stress levels of those who took advantage of the parks steadily dropped.[3]

When you combine nature and new experiences, you're tapping into a powerful source of strength and vitality. Hiking, biking, roller blading, kayaking, and skiing are just a few of the many ways to enjoy fresh air, exercise, and, for some of you, new experiences. Those of you who are already active outdoors can try hiking or bik-ing new trails and skiing new slopes. And because you're working out and feeling stronger, these activities will be more fun because you'll feel more capable of doing them.

 Take advantage of nearby parks, trails, and waterways. Make it fun by giving yourself some milestones. Make it a goal to hike or bike one trail in every county in your state or to visit every national park over the next decade.

Experiment with food and cooking

You don't have to climb Mount Everest to be adventurous. Experi-menting in the kitchen is full of adventure (and just a little safer). If you've fallen into a rut with the meals you cook and where you eat them, it's time to break new ground in the food department. Try some of these novel ideas:

- Take a cooking class.
- Start a cookbook club.
- Commit to inviting people over for dinner at least once a month.
- Make a different ethnic dish every week.
- Host a cooking party.
- Try a veggie that's not currently in your vocabulary. Jicama, a crunchy veggie, makes for a perfect healthy snack.

- Spiralize beets and see if you like them any better than sliced beets.
- Buy a small appliance you're curious about, an air fryer or an Instant Pot, for instance.
- Paint your kitchen, resurface your cabinets, or redecorate entirely (especially after you declutter!).
- Buy a fresh set of kitchen towels.
- Start an indoor herb garden.
- Plant an indoor or outdoor vegetable garden.
- Experiment with different spices, herbs, and recipes.
- Try a new restaurant.
- Invite someone you don't typically eat with to lunch or dinner.

I'm sure you can come up with many other ways to shake things up. Think of things you've always wanted to do or try. Even the smallest changes, such as testing out a new recipe or scheduling daily walks in the park, can challenge you to stretch your horizons. Write them down. Promise yourself you'll do them. Then, make them happen.

Wedge of Wisdom

Many of my clients are in New York City, where we are surrounded by concrete and tall buildings. Some of my clients don't even think to get out in nature and exercise outdoors until I start talking about it. Mary Ann disliked the gym. She would join and go for a month until she got busy and bored. When I suggested she take advantage of nature and exercise outdoors (weather permitting), she tried it and became hooked. She didn't enjoy running on a treadmill, but she loved jogging and walking outdoors. Doing something she enjoyed helped her stick to her food plan and lose those last 10 pounds she'd been hanging on to.

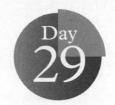

Pursue Your Passion

> The meaning of life is to find your gift. The purpose of life
> is to give it away.
>
> —David Viscott

Ever look up at the clock, shocked to see that hours have passed and it felt like moments? You were likely doing something you're passionate about.

Passion is an intense, enthusiastic drive. A calling. When we're doing something we feel passionate about, we're so absorbed we lose track of time. We're in the zone, that mental state where we're most productive, with laser-sharp focus and clarity. We forget ourselves and everything else. We're connected, it seems, to something bigger than ourselves. Athletes and creatives talk about it a lot. But almost everyone has had the experience, even if for brief moments. The theory is that, when you're in the zone, you're doing something related to your purpose, or the gift you're meant to share with the world.

I subscribe to the idea that everyone has a passion to share, and I encourage you to pursue yours, if you haven't already. A researcher at the University of Quebec found that when we regularly engage in activities we like or love, we improve our well-being.[1] We're more

RATE YOUR PASSION

Feeling passionate is a fine line, or a narrow path, between anxiety and boredom, depending on our ability to handle the task and whether it's challenging enough or overwhelming. If what we're doing is way outside of our skill level, we become anxious. If the activity is too easy for us, we get bored. "The zone" is a sweet spot where the right amount of skill and challenge meet and energize us.[2]

satisfied, feel empowered, and experience greater self-awareness and self-confidence. Without passion, we can feel a void, or an emptiness we long to fill.

Ask yourself, *What's my passion? How has this program helped me to develop a passion for good health or working out? Has my weight loss inspired any new passions? Or was I waiting to find my passion till after the weight was lost?* My hope is that the Program outlined in this book has inspired you to explore all your passions in addition to living a healthy lifestyle even mini-passions, such as taking a cooking class, getting out on the golf course, or digging into your garden. Home in on your passion and go for it!

Bite-Sized Goodie About 25 percent of Americans claim to have a strong sense of purpose and meaning in their lives. Another 40 percent are neutral or say they do not have purpose.[3] Research increasingly suggests that a sense of purpose is important for a meaningful life—but also for a healthy life. Studies show that having purpose improves sleep and lowers the risk of dementia, stroke, and heart attack. People who find meaning in life are also more likely to take care of their physical health by scheduling preventive checkups, such as mammograms and colonoscopies.[4]

Find your passion

Passion doesn't always just come to us. Sometimes we have to actively search for it. And it's not always obvious to us, especially if we let fear take over. Some of us have to get out and stretch our horizons to come across something we feel passionate about. Think about what you're drawn to or things you've always wanted to do. Don't judge these thoughts—or your ability to accomplish them (that's fear in disguise). Rather, think of how you can build your skills in this area. If you've always desired to act, go to plays, take an acting class, read about famous actors. And then practice. If you're just beginning, start small. You don't need to think about moving to Hollywood or getting a talent agent. That kind of pressure might throw you out of the zone. Do what inspires you. When you're ready, we'll see you on the silver screen.

Passion can be applied to anything in life, including cooking, hiking, accounting, and studying. Passion doesn't require a paycheck. You can volunteer or make works of art for yourself. Think of your desires and your skill levels and go from there. Just make it meaningful to you, make it challenging enough, and don't bite off more than you can chew. When you're in the zone, you'll know.

Wedge of Wisdom

Patty always wanted to run a half marathon but was too out of shape and overweight. She started walking and doing light jogs. She knew that the health club she belonged to had a running group. One day Patty struck up a conversation with the lead runner, who assured her that the group accepted people from all levels. Reluctantly, Patty joined the group for an evening run. She was the last and slowest runner. But it didn't matter. Everyone in the group would run back to her and swoop her up so she wasn't left behind. She felt inspired (and even loved) by their encouragement and kept running with the group. After a year, she was keeping up with one or two other runners in the group, had lost 40 pounds, and was ready to join the club's group training for marathons.

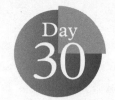

Start Each
Day Anew

Create the highest, grandest vision possible for your life,
because you become what you believe.

—Oprah Winfrey

In Day #17: Eat Mindfully (page 162), we discussed being fully
present and eating in the moment. We put all our attention on our
food and the act of eating it. We learned that eating mindfully can
lead to eating less, enjoying our food more, and losing weight. This
chapter applies the practice of mindfulness to everything you do.
Living in the present moment has many benefits beyond weight loss.

Some benefits of living in the present

Harvard researchers found that the happiest people thought about
what they were doing at the moment. It didn't matter what they were
doing. They could have been shoveling snow or on a cruise. The
mere act of fully being there for it (without judgment) was all that
mattered. Syncing our thoughts and actions makes us happy.[1] And
happy people live longer.[2] One of the benefits to living in the moment,
then, is a longer, fuller life. Other benefits include the following:

You stop thinking about your performance. You don't wake up every morning so you can jump on the scale. One day, you find you've lost 10 pounds and note how happy you feel. You don't judge. You don't obsess. You don't worry. You free yourself to enjoy each moment—the collection of which is also known as your life.

You stop worrying. Worry is always about something that might happen in the future. And it's stressful. The only time you can actually do something about your worry is in the present moment. Rather than worry, you can calmly do something now to prevent your impending disaster so it doesn't happen. If it's out of your control, you can accept that fact.

You accept everything without judgment. If it bothers you, you don't run away but move toward it, or embrace it. Acceptance is the first step toward change.

You take time to just breathe. When I get stressed, I stop and take a few deep breaths. This brings me back to the moment. Most of us don't worry about our next breath, much less think about it. When we focus on our breath, it brings our awareness to what's happening in the moment.

You're in the zone. Instead of tracking time, you flow with it.

You engage with others. Honestly and fully.

You escape your monkey thoughts, or the endless chatter that takes place in the mind. Stepping away from these thoughts gives you calm, peace, and clarity. You make better decisions.

TIPS FOR HOW TO BE PRESENT

Focus on one thing at a time.

Be deliberate and methodical.

Fully listen to the person who's speaking to you. Look into his or her eyes.

Eat slowly and savor every bite.

Bite-Sized Goodie According to Harvard researchers, we spend almost half our time doing one thing and thinking about another.[3]

Start each day with a clean slate

I like to start each day with a clean slate. Every night before going to bed, I rewind my day. If I offended someone, did I apologize? If I felt wronged by another, did I forgive him or her? If you're in contact with enough people every day, your list of resentments can get pretty long pretty quickly. Rather than carry around all this baggage, I try to dump it at the end of each day. I don't want it affecting what I do or how I behave the next day. And, figuratively speaking, I do not want to lug around years' worth of heavy baggage. A clean slate frees me up to be present. And I'm happier because of it.

Finally Full, Finally Slim is about more than the number on the scale and eating thoughtful portions of healthy foods. Leading a full life by doing what you love and being the person you want to be is nourishment as well. Living life to the fullest leaves you feeling satisfied all around, and you're more likely to maintain your healthy weight.

Whether you've lost weight by following the Plan or are contemplating whether to start, I encourage you to focus on what you can do now. Worrying about past diet failures or fearing that you will regain any weight lost puts you in the past and the future. We can't change the past. And we can't live in the future. We can only put our energy into the present moment.

My hope is that you'll use all the tools you've learned in this program and incorporate them into your life moving forward. Together, they really do help you start each day anew, so that you are finally full and finally slim.

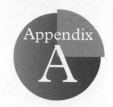

Comprehensive Food List with Serving Sizes

These lists are more comprehensive than the lists found in the Finally Full, Finally Slim Portion Plan (page 18).

VEGETABLES (NONSTARCHY)

Unlimited; at least 3 servings daily

1 cup raw or ½ cup cooked

Alfalfa sprouts	Eggplant
Artichokes	Fennel
Asparagus	Green beans
Bamboo shoots	Greens (collards, kale,
Bean sprouts	mustard, turnip)
Beets	Kohlrabi
Broccoli	Leeks
Brussels sprouts	Mushrooms
Carrots	Okra
Cauliflower	Onions
Celery	Pea pods
Cucumber	Peppers (red, yellow, green)

Radishes

Salad greens (arugula, endive, escarole, assorted lettuce)

Scallions

Snow peas

Spaghetti squash

Spinach

Sugar snap peas

Summer squash (yellow or zucchini)

Tomatoes

Water chestnuts

Watercress

Salsa, ½ cup

Tomato sauce, tomato puree, ½ cup

Tomato juice, 1 cup (8 ounces)

Vegetable juice, 1 cup (8 ounces)

Vegetable soup, 1 cup (8 ounces)

GO FOR IT: *All veggies, especially a colorful assortment; low-sodium vegetable juices and soups*

PUT A LID ON IT: *Canned or frozen vegetables with added sauces or other ingredients*

FRUITS

Unlimited whole fruits; at least 2 servings daily

Apple, 1

Applesauce, unsweetened, ½ cup

Apricots, fresh, 4 whole

Banana, 1

Berries (blackberries, blueberries, raspberries, strawberries), 1 cup

Canned fruit, unsweetened, 1 cup

Cantaloupe, ½ melon or 1 cup cubed

Cherries, fresh, 1 cup

Clementines, 2

Dried fruit (apricots, dates, figs, peaches, prunes), ¼ cup;
    1 small box of raisins

Figs, fresh, 2

Fruit juice (orange, grapefruit, cranberry), 4 ounces

Fruit smoothie (use no more than 1 cup mixed fruit), ice water,
    and ice as desired, 10–12 ounces

Fruit salad (mixed fruits), 1 cup

Grapefruit, ½

Grapes, 1 cup

Honeydew, 1 cup cubed

Kiwifruit, 2

Mango, ½, or 1 cup cubed

Nectarine, 1

Orange, 1

Papaya, ½, or 1 cup cubed

Peach, 1

Pear, 1

Pomegranate seeds, ½ cup

Persimmon, ½, or 1 cup cubed

Pineapple, fresh, 1 cup cubed

Plums, 2

Tangerines, 2

Watermelon, 1 cup cubed

GO FOR IT: *All fresh or frozen fruits*

PUT A LID ON IT: *Limit your intake of fruit juice and dried fruit; skip canned or frozen fruits in syrup; limit fruit smoothies to one a day (use up to 1 cup fruit)*

STARCHES (GRAINS AND STARCHY VEGETABLES)

4–6 servings daily

Starchy Vegetables

Cassava (yucca), ½ cup cooked

Corn, 1 ear, or ½ cup cooked

Legumes* (black-eyed peas, black beans, chickpeas/garbanzo beans, green peas, kidney beans, lentils, lima beans, pinto beans, snap peas, snow peas, split peas, white beans), ½ cup cooked

  *NOTE: These can also be counted as a meat alternative. Do not count in both groups.

Parsnip, ½ cup cooked

Plantain, ½ cup cooked

Potato, baked with skin, ½, 3–4 ounces, or ½ cup

Potato, boiled, ½ cup

Rutabaga, ½ cup cooked

Sweet potato, yam, baked, ½, 3–4 ounces, or ½ cup

Winter squash (butternut, acorn, pumpkin), 1 cup cooked

Whole Grains

Amaranth, ½ cup cooked

Barley, ½ cup cooked

Bread slice, whole grain (whole wheat, rye, oat, sprouted grain), 1 ounce

Breadsticks, whole grain, 3 (about 4½ inches)

Brown rice, ½ cup cooked

Bulgur (tabouli), ½ cup cooked

Cereal, whole grain, ½ cup cooked (¼ cup uncooked or 1 packet)

  Buckwheat groats

  Cracked wheat

    Oat bran

    Oatmeal

    Wheatena

Cereal, ready-to-eat (cold), unsweetened, whole grain, 1 ounce

    Brown rice cereal, 1 cup

    Flakes (bran, corn, oat), 1 cup

    Oat rings (Cheerios), 1 cup

    Puffed wheat or puffed brown rice, 2 cups

    Shredded Wheat (1 biscuit)

    Spoon Size Shredded Wheat, ½ cup

    Low-fat granola, nuggets, muesli, ¼ cup

Cereal or granola bar, whole grain, 1, 1 ounce

Couscous, whole wheat, ½ cup cooked

Crackers, whole-grain varieties, 1 ounce, 2–3 large, 5–6 small
    (see product food label for exact number of crackers)

    Flatbreads, whole grain, 2–3, rye (Ryvita) or Kavli crisps

    Mini crackers, 10 (Mary's Gone Crackers)

English muffin, whole grain, sprouted grain, ½ (about 1 ounce)

Farro, ½ cup cooked

Kasha (buckwheat groats), ½ cup cooked

Matzo, whole wheat, 1 sheet

Millet, ½ cup cooked

Muffin, whole grain, 1 ounce (about ¼ muffin)

Pancake, whole-grain varieties, 1 (1 ounce, or about 4 inches in
    diameter)

Pasta, whole wheat, ½ cup cooked

    Legume pasta (black bean, lentil, chickpea), ½ cup cooked

Pita, whole wheat, 1 (1 ounce, or about 4 inches in diameter)

    1 large pita, 2 ounces, is 2 servings

Popcorn, air-popped (no fat added), 3 cups

Pretzels, whole wheat or oat bran, 1 ounce, or ¾ cup
    (1 small bag)

Puffed grain cakes (brown rice and quinoa blend), 1 ounce, about 4

Quinoa, ½ cup cooked

Rice (brown rice, wild rice), ½ cup cooked

Rice cakes, 2 regular, or 6 mini

Rice noodles (brown rice), ½ cup cooked

Soba noodles, ½ cup cooked

Sorghum, ½ cup cooked

Tortilla, whole wheat, 1 ounce (7 inches in diameter)

   1 large tortilla, 2 ounces, is 2 servings

Waffle, whole-grain varieties, 1 (1 ounce or about 4 inches square)

Wheat germ, 3 tablespoons

White-Flour Products

Bagel, 1 ounce (about ¼ bagel)

Bread slice, cereal, pancakes, pita, tortilla, waffles, white-bread varieties (follow serving sizes of whole-grain varieties)

Corn taco shells, 2

Crackers, 1 ounce (see product food label for exact number of crackers)

   2–3 large crackers (size of graham crackers, bread sticks)

   5–6 small crackers (size of saltines)

   24 oyster crackers

Muffin, 1 ounce (about ¼ muffin)

Pasta (spaghetti, macaroni, lasagna noodles), ½ cup cooked

Pretzels, 1 ounce (¾ cup)

   1 Bavarian Baldie

   2 pretzel rods

   9 three-ring twists

   20 mini-twists

   48 sticks

Rice, white, ½ cup cooked

GO FOR IT: *Whole-grain breads and cereals (whole wheat, rye, oat); cooked cereal, such as oatmeal; brown rice, quinoa, kasha, bulgur, barley, wild rice; all starchy vegetables such as sweet potatoes, beans, and winter squash; and legumes such as lentils, chickpeas, and split peas*

PUT A LID ON IT: *White-flour products, such as white bread, pasta, bagels, crackers, muffins, pretzels, white rice; cereals with added sugar; and, of course, skip the oversized bread products*

BE MINDFUL: *"Single-serve" items such as muffins, bagels, scones, street pretzels, and knishes can be up to 5 or 6 servings!*

Brown bread does not mean whole-wheat bread. Multigrain does not mean whole grain. Read the label and look for the word "whole" in the ingredients list.

FISH, POULTRY, MEAT, AND MEAT ALTERNATIVES

2–3 servings daily (6–9 ounces)

Fish, Poultry, Meat

3–4 ounces cooked*
*NOTE: 4 ounces raw yields 3 ounces cooked
Beef, lamb, veal, pork (choose lean varieties)
Chicken
Cornish hen
Fish (salmon, tuna, filet of sole, halibut, flounder, red
    snapper, striped bass, haddock, trout, cod, sea bass)
Game (buffalo, venison)
Liver
Seafood (shrimp, scallops, lobster)
Turkey

Meat Alternatives

Bean (split pea, white bean) or lentil soup, 1 cup

Cooked beans and legumes, 1 cup cooked

Edamame, ½ cup

Eggs, 2; egg substitute, ½ cup

Egg whites, 4–6

Hummus (and other bean dips), ½ cup

Veggie/bean burger, 1, 3 ounces

Soy burger, 1, 3 ounces

Tofu or tempeh, 1 cup

*NOTE: 1 ounce meat, fish, or poultry = 1 egg, or 2 egg whites, or ½ cup legumes

GO FOR IT: *Fish, skinless poultry, legumes, tempeh, eggs, lean and extra-lean cuts of beef, veal, and lamb (USDA Select or Choice grades, trimmed, such as round, sirloin, and flank steak; tenderloin; roast; T-bone)*

PUT A LID ON IT: *High-fat cuts of beef, lamb, and veal; processed sandwich meats such as salami, bologna; sausage; hot dogs; bacon; spareribs*

BE MINDFUL: *Include a little bit of protein with each meal (with the emphasis on "little").*

Include fish at least twice a week.

Try to incorporate one meat alternative daily.

Limit red meat to no more than once or twice a week.

Don't exceed more than 2 servings of fish, poultry, or meat (6 ounces cooked) at one sitting.

DAIRY

2–3 servings daily

Fat-Free and Low-Fat Dairy

Buttermilk, fat-free or low fat, 1 cup

Cheese, Parmesan, grated, 3–4 tablespoons

Cottage cheese, fat-free or low fat, ½ cup

Dry nonfat milk, evaporated milk, ½ cup

Hard cheese, part skim, or low fat, 2 slices, 1½–2 ounces

Hoop cheese, pot cheese, ½ cup

Ice milk, 1 cup

Kefir, fat-free or low fat, 1 cup

Milk, fat-free or low fat (1 percent), 1 cup (8 fluid ounces)

Ricotta cheese, part skim, ½ cup

Shredded cheese, part skim, ⅓ cup

Yogurt, fat-free or low fat, 1 cup (6–8 fluid ounces)

Whole-Milk Dairy

Hard cheese, whole-milk varieties, 2 slices, 1½–2 ounces

Kefir, whole milk, 1 cup

Ricotta cheese, whole milk, ½ cup

Shredded cheese, ⅓ cup

Whole milk, 1 cup (8 fluid ounces)

Yogurt, whole milk, 1 cup (6–8 fluid ounces)

Milk Swaps

Almond milk and other nut milks, unsweetened, calcium and
vitamin D fortified, 1 cup (8 fluid ounces)

Coconut milk, unsweetened, calcium and vitamin D fortified, 1
cup (8 fluid ounces)

Oat milk, unsweetened, calcium and vitamin D fortified, 1 cup
(8 fluid ounces)

Soy milk, unsweetened, calcium and vitamin D fortified, 1 cup
(8 fluid ounces)

Yogurt, dairy-free, 1 cup (6–8 fluid ounces)

GO FOR IT: *Fat-free, low-fat, and part-skim dairy products; unsweetened, calcium- and vitamin D–fortified nut milks*

PUT A LID ON IT: *Whole-milk dairy and sugar-sweetened milk and milk swaps*

BE MINDFUL: *Dairy is a good source of protein and an easy and healthful snack.*

FATS

2–3 servings daily

Healthy Fats

Avocado, ¼ cup (¼–⅓ avocado, depending on size)

Nuts (almonds, walnuts, peanuts, cashews, pistachios, pecans, pine nuts, Brazil nuts), 1 ounce (about ¼ cup)

Nut butter (peanut butter, almond butter, cashew butter, seed butter), 1 tablespoon (3 teaspoons)

Oil (extra-virgin olive oil, grape-seed oil, canola oil, nut/seed oil, vegetable oil), 1 tablespoon (3 teaspoons)

Olives, 12–15 medium

Salad dressing (olive-oil based), 2 tablespoons

Salad dressing, reduced fat, 2 tablespoons

Seeds (sesame, sunflower, pumpkin), 1 ounce (about ¼ cup)

Tahini paste, 1 tablespoon

Ground flaxseeds, 2–3 tablespoons

Chia seeds, 2–3 tablespoons

Hemp seeds, 2–3 tablespoons

Less-Healthy Fats

Butter, 1 tablespoon

Coconut, shredded, 3 tablespoons

Coconut oil, 1 tablespoon

Cream, 2 tablespoons

Cream cheese, 1 tablespoon

Margarine, 1 tablespoon

Mayonnaise, 1 tablespoon

Salad dressing (creamy), 1 tablespoon

Sour cream, 2 tablespoons

GO FOR IT: *Healthy fats such as avocado oil, olive oil, canola oil, soybean oil, most vegetable oils, tahini, avocado, olives, nuts, nut butters, seeds*

PUT A LID ON IT: *Less-healthy fats such as butter, coconut oil, cream cheese, margarine, mayonnaise, creamy salad dressing*

BE MINDFUL: *Fats contain more than double the calories of carbohydrates and protein, so be sure to watch portion sizes. Even healthy fats contain calories.*

TREATS AND SWEETS

0–2 servings daily

Alcoholic beverages

Beer, 12 ounces

Spirits (vodka, whiskey, gin, rum, tequila), 1½ ounces

Wine, 5–6 ounces

Cakes and cookies, 1 ounce

Biscotti, 1

Cake sliver, 1

Cookies, 2 small (2 inches)

Cupcake, mini, 1

Graham crackers, 4 squares

Pie, ⅓ cup

Candies and sweets, ¼ cup unless otherwise indicated

Chocolate

Bite-sized, fun-size, mini, or trick-or-treat-size bar, 1

Hershey's Kisses, 4

M&M'S candies, ¼ cup

York Peppermint Patties, small, 2

Flavored popcorn, ½ cup

Fruit Roll-Up, 1

Hard candy, 3

Licorice, 2 twists

Lollipop, 1 Tootsie Pop or Charms Blow Pop

Peanut brittle, 1 ounce

Tootsie Roll, 3 small

Chips (corn chips, potato chips, tortilla chips), ½ cup (if you
want to count: 15 corn chips, 10 potato chips, 10 tortilla
chips)

Fried foods

French fries, ½ cup

Fried onion rings, ½ cup

Frozen treats

Ice cream, ½ cup

Italian ice, ½ cup

Frozen yogurt, ½ cup

Low-fat or fat-free ice cream, ½ cup

Popsicle, 1 (frozen fruit pop, fudge pop)

Sorbet, ½ cup

Fruit and nut / energy bar, 1 ounce, 1 KIND mini bar, ½ Clif
Bar, ½ Luna Bar

Gravies and sauces, 1–2 tablespoons

Sugar, honey, jelly, maple syrup, 1–2 tablespoons

GO FOR IT: *Eat only what you love. Plan for a treat. Choose single servings.*

PUT A LID ON IT: *Large, sugary beverages; foods you tend to overeat; munching straight from jumbo bags*

BE MINDFUL: *Plan for a treat. Legalize it.*

WATER

Drink 64 ounces daily (eight 8-ounce glasses): water, seltzer, sparkling water, herbal tea.

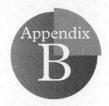

Portion Plans

Following are several sample meal plans based on different Finally Full, Finally Slim Numbers (see page 21). The plans list meals and ingredients but not cooking directions. If you are unsure how to make any given meal, look up a similar recipe and apply the same cooking procedure.

Portion Plan A

Finally Full, Finally Slim Number (the number of servings you should have based on factors such as gender, age, and activity level; see page 21):

3+ servings Vegetables (Nonstarchy)

2+ servings Fruits

4 servings Starches (Grains and Starchy Vegetables)

2 servings Fish, Poultry, Meat, and Meat Alternatives

2 servings Dairy

2 servings Fats

▶ Breakfast

Greek yogurt parfait

1 cup plain or vanilla low-fat Greek yogurt or almond milk yogurt	1 DAIRY
1 cup mixed blueberries and blackberries	1 FRUIT
1 teaspoon flaxseeds	
Cinnamon and vanilla for flavor	

Coffee or tea with fat-free or low-fat milk (optional)

▶ Lunch

Black bean burrito bowl with farro

1 cup farro	2 STARCHES
½ cup black beans	½ MEAT ALTERNATIVE
½ cup chopped bell peppers	½ VEGETABLE
½ cup cherry tomatoes	½ VEGETABLE
1 cup spinach	1 VEGETABLE
¼ cup salsa	½ VEGETABLE
1½ ounces shredded part-skim mozzarella cheese	1 DAIRY
Balsamic vinaigrette dressing, 1 tablespoon	½ FAT

▶ Snack

Apple with 1–2 teaspoons peanut butter	1 FRUIT; ½ FAT

▶ Dinner

Vegetable soup, 8–10 ounces	1 VEGETABLE

Grilled salmon with roasted sweet potatoes and Brussels sprouts

5 ounces salmon	1½ FISH
1½ cups roasted Brussels sprouts and cauliflower	3 VEGETABLES
1 cup roasted sweet potatoes	2 STARCHES
1 tablespoon olive oil for roasting	1 FAT

❱ Snack

1 cup frozen grapes	1 FRUIT

Portion Plan B

Finally Full, Finally Slim Number (the number of servings you should have based on factors such as gender, age, and activity level; see page 21):

3+ servings Vegetables (Nonstarchy)
2+ servings Fruits
4 servings Starches (Grains and Starchy Vegetables)
2 servings Fish, Poultry, Meat, and Meat Alternatives
2 servings Dairy
2 servings Fats

❱ Breakfast

Apple-berry oatmeal

1 cup cooked oatmeal	2 STARCHES
½ cup blueberries and ½ apple	1 FRUIT
1 cup low-fat milk, fat-free milk, or unsweetened vanilla almond milk	1 DAIRY
Cinnamon, vanilla extract to taste	
1 teaspoon chia seeds or hemp seeds	

Coffee or tea with fat-free or low-fat milk (optional)

If you prefer to mix oatmeal with water, you can add low-fat Greek yogurt. To boost flavor, add the fruit to the uncooked oatmeal.

▶ Lunch

Salad entrée

2 cups mixed lettuce—romaine, Bibb, radicchio	2 VEGETABLES
1 cup chopped carrots, cucumbers, tomato, and peppers	1 VEGETABLE
½ cup chickpeas	½ MEAT ALTERNATIVE
Sliced hard-boiled egg	½ MEAT ALTERNATIVE
1 tablespoon honey mustard vinaigrette	½ FAT

▶ Snack

Frozen banana

1 banana	1 FRUIT
1–2 teaspoons peanut butter	½ FAT

Peel the banana, add the peanut butter, and sprinkle on some cinnamon (optional). Put in a baggie and freeze for at least 1 hour.

▶ Dinner

Vegetable soup (8–10 ounces)	1 VEGETABLE

Grilled chicken with vegetables

4 ounces grilled chicken breast	1 POULTRY
1 tablespoon barbecue or teriyaki sauce (optional)	
1½ cups sautéed broccoli and snap peas	3 VEGETABLES
1 cup roasted butternut squash	1 STARCH
1 tablespoon olive oil to sauté	1 FAT

▶ Snack

3 cups air-popped popcorn	1 STARCH

Fruit smoothie

1 cup raspberries, strawberries, and blueberries (fresh or frozen)	1 FRUIT
1 cup fat-free milk, low-fat milk, or your favorite unsweetened milk swap	1 DAIRY
1 tablespoon peanut powder and ¼ teaspoon vanilla or cocoa powder, to taste (optional)	
1 cup crushed ice or 5–6 ice cubes	

Portion Plan C

Finally Full, Finally Slim Number (the number of servings you should have based on factors such as gender, age, and activity level; see page 21):

3+ servings Vegetables (Nonstarchy)

2+ servings Fruits

4–5 servings Starches (Grains and Starchy Vegetables)

3 servings Fish, Poultry, Meat, and Meat Alternatives

2 servings Dairy

2½ servings Fats

1 serving Treats and Sweets

▶ Breakfast

Avocado toast cheese melt

1–2 slices sprouted whole-grain toast	1–2 STARCHES
¼ cup avocado, mashed	1 FAT
Sliced tomato, fresh parsley	1 VEGETABLE
Part-skim Swiss cheese, 2 slices (1½ ounces)	1 DAIRY
½ grapefruit or 1 orange	1 FRUIT
Coffee or tea with fat-free or low-fat milk (optional)	

▶ Lunch

Grilled or canned salmon, acorn squash, and arugula salad

2 cups arugula	2 VEGETABLES
½ acorn squash (1 cup)	1 STARCH
3 ounces salmon	1 FISH
½ cup pomegranate seeds	1 FRUIT
½ cup white beans	½ MEAT ALTERNATIVE
1 tablespoon balsamic vinaigrette dressing	½ FAT

▶ Snack

Hummus, ¼ cup	½ MEAT ALTERNATIVE
1 cup jicama, baby carrots, and sliced red pepper	1 VEGETABLE

▶ Dinner

Zucchini noodles (zoodles) and pasta with turkey meatballs or grilled tempeh

3 ounces turkey meatballs or grilled tempeh	1 POULTRY OR MEAT ALTERNATIVE
1 cup zoodles (cooked)	2 VEGETABLES
1 cup whole-wheat pasta or soba noodles	2 STARCHES
½ cup tomato sauce	1 VEGETABLE
1 cup sautéed cauliflower and broccoli	2 VEGETABLES
1 tablespoon olive oil	1 FAT
2 tablespoons fresh chopped parsley, oregano, and garlic (optional)	

▶ Snack

1 baked apple	1 FRUIT
½ cup cottage cheese topped with nutmeg and cinnamon	1 DAIRY
1 teaspoon chopped walnuts (optional)	
1 piece (½ ounce) dark chocolate–almond bark (70 percent cocoa)	1 TREATS AND SWEETS

Portion Plan D

Finally Full, Finally Slim Number (the number of servings you should have based on factors such as gender, age, and activity level; see page 21):

   3+ servings Vegetables (Nonstarchy)
   2+ servings Fruits

5 servings Starches (Grains and Starchy Vegetables)

2½ servings Fish, Poultry, Meat, and Meat Alternatives

2 servings Dairy

3 servings Fats

1 serving Treats and Sweets

▶ Breakfast

Spinach tomato omelet

2-egg omelet or 4–6 egg whites or ½ cup egg whites or Egg Beaters	1 MEAT ALTERNATIVE
1 cup spinach and tomatoes	1 VEGETABLE
Black pepper, oregano to taste	
Olive oil to coat pan	½ FAT
1 slice whole-grain or Ezekiel toast with 2 tablespoons avocado	1 STARCH; ½ FAT
1 cup watermelon	1 FRUIT
Coffee or tea with fat-free or low-fat milk (optional)	

▶ Lunch

Kale, lentil, and quinoa salad

1 cup kale	1 VEGETABLE
1 cup shaved Brussels sprouts	1 VEGETABLE
2 tablespoons olive oil–based dressing	1 FAT
1 cup quinoa	2 STARCHES
½ cup lentils	½ MEAT ALTERNATIVE
3–4 tablespoons Parmesan cheese	1 DAIRY

▶ Snack

Yogurt berry parfait

1 cup yogurt or dairy-free yogurt	1 DAIRY
1 cup raspberries and blueberries	1 FRUIT
1 teaspoon hemp or chia seeds	

▶ Dinner

5 ounces red wine (optional)	1 TREATS AND SWEETS

Chicken or tuna and vegetable stir-fry

3–4 ounces chicken breast or fresh tuna, cubed	1 POULTRY
1½ cups sautéed asparagus, carrots, and broccoli	3 VEGETABLES
1 tablespoon olive oil or sesame oil	1 FAT
Garlic, ginger, low-sodium soy sauce to taste	
1 cup wild rice	2 STARCHES

▶ Snack

Rainbow fruit salad

1 cup kiwifruit, watermelon, blackberries, and pomegranate seeds (or your favorite colorful fruit concoction)	1 FRUIT
2 teaspoons slivered almonds (optional)	

Mix and Match Portion Plans

Below are thirty mix-and-match breakfast/brunch and lunch/dinner options, along with snacks. Mix and match these options to create a variety of portion-perfect meals. Adjust the serving sizes to meet your specific Finally Full, Finally Slim Number (see page 21).

Breakfast and Brunch Options

Breakfast does not have to be eaten as soon as you wake up. Rushing to work in the morning? Don't stress out about food. It's fine to eat it when you get to work or even midmorning. Some simple breakfast ideas can also be prepared in advance. If you are not much of a breakfast eater, choose a breakfast on the lighter side.

▶ *Peanut butter berry overnight oats*

1 cup fresh or frozen blueberries and strawberries
1 teaspoon hemp seeds, chia seeds, or ground flaxseeds
½ cup old-fashioned or quick whole-grain oats
¾ cup fat-free milk or unsweetened vanilla almond milk
2 teaspoons peanut butter (or nut butter of choice)
¼ teaspoon pure vanilla extract
Cinnamon to taste

▶ *Greek yogurt parfait*

1 cup plain or vanilla low-fat Greek yogurt or almond milk yogurt
¼ cup pomegranate seeds
½ apple, chopped
1 tablespoon slivered almonds or hemp seeds (Manitoba Harvest)

▶ *Spinach, mushroom, and artichoke omelet*

2 eggs, or 4–6 egg whites (½ cup), or egg substitute (½ cup)
½ cup raw spinach
¼ cup sliced artichoke hearts
¼ cup mushrooms
Olive oil to coat pan or mug

(You can make a veggie egg scramble in an oversized mug.)

1 slice sprouted-grain or whole-wheat toast
2 tablespoons (1 thin schmear) avocado spread

▶ Cottage cheese berry crunch

½ cup low-fat cottage cheese or pot cheese
1 cup mixed berries or melon (cantaloupe, honeydew, watermelon)
½ cup cereal for crunch (Barbara's Puffins, Cheerios, or whole-grain cereal of
    choice), or 1 muffin top (2 ounces, such as VitaTops)

▶ Avocado toast with egg and cherry tomatoes

1 slice whole-grain bread
2 tablespoons (6 teaspoons) mashed avocado
1 egg, sunny-side up or hard-boiled
½ cup cherry tomatoes

▶ Quinoa breakfast bowl

1 cup quinoa, cooked
1 cup fat-free, low-fat milk, or unsweetened milk swap
Cinnamon and nutmeg to taste
1 sliced pear
1 teaspoon flaxseeds or hemp seeds

▶ Banola—peanut butter, banana, and granola

1 banana, peeled
1 tablespoon peanut butter
¼ cup sprinkling of no-sugar-added granola (optional)

(Freeze for at least 30 minutes before serving.)

▶ Yogurt with blackberries and pistachios

1 cup plain or vanilla low-fat Greek yogurt or dairy-free yogurt
1 cup blackberries
2 tablespoons chopped pistachios
Cinnamon and vanilla extract to taste

▶ Whole-grain waffle with almond butter and berries

1 whole-grain waffle
2 teaspoons almond butter
1 cup strawberries

▶ *Ready-to-eat whole-grain cereal with berries*

1 cup unsweetened Cheerios or Barbara's Puffins, or your favorite whole-grain
    cereal with at least 3 grams fiber
1 cup blueberries and raspberries
1 tablespoon crushed walnuts

▶ *Blueberry-pear smoothie*

1 cup low-fat or fat-free milk or 6 ounces yogurt
½ cup fresh or frozen blueberries
½ pear, or 1 kiwifruit
½ cup spinach
1 tablespoon flaxseeds or chia seeds
1 tablespoon peanut powder
1 cup crushed ice or 5–6 ice cubes

▶ *Homemade apple cinnamon oatmeal*

⅓ cup steel-cut oats, dry
1 cup unsweetened vanilla almond milk, fat-free milk, low-fat milk, or water
1 apple, diced (add to oatmeal before cooking)
Cinnamon and vanilla to taste

▶ *Chia seed pudding*

¼ cup chia seeds
1 cup unsweetened vanilla almond milk or your favorite milk swap
1 cup mixed berries (raspberries and blueberries)
Cinnamon and vanilla

(Add ingredients to a mason jar or a container with a lid, mix, and chill for 1 hour.)

▶ *English muffin breakfast sandwich*

1 sprouted whole-grain English muffin or whole-wheat English muffin
1 hard-boiled egg or 2 ounces sliced, grilled tempeh
½ tomato, sliced
¼ medium avocado

▶ *Strawberry-chocolate ricotta toast*

1 slice whole-grain toast
½ cup part-skim ricotta or pot cheese
1 cup strawberries, sliced
1 teaspoon cacao nibs (optional)

(Bake all ingredients together for several minutes to boost flavor.)

❱ *Baked pumpkin oatmeal*

½ cup rolled oats, dry
¼ cup pumpkin puree
½ cup unsweetened vanilla almond milk or your favorite milk swap
¼ teaspoon vanilla extract
Cinnamon, vanilla, pumpkin pie spice
1 plum, sliced

❱ *Tomato, cheese, and edamame toast*

1 slice sprouted-grain or whole-grain bread, toasted
1 ounce shredded mozzarella cheese
6 sliced cherry tomatoes
¼ cup edamame
Drizzle of olive oil

❱ *Toasted sweet potato with hard-boiled egg and Israeli salad*

1 medium sweet potato, sliced and toasted
1 hard-boiled egg, or ½ cup edamame
1 cup Israeli salad—chopped tomatoes, cucumber, and onions
Drizzle of olive oil and lemon (optional)

❱ *Apricot smoothie*

2 fresh apricots, diced
4–6 ounces fat-free or low-fat milk, or 1 container (6 ounces) low-fat vanilla
    Greek yogurt
1–2 tablespoons peanut powder
Vanilla, cinnamon (optional)
1 tablespoon hemp or chia seeds
1 cup crushed ice or 5–6 ice cubes

(Add iced water as desired for a thinner consistency.)

❱ *Very berry yogurt parfait*

1 cup fat-free or low-fat plain or vanilla Greek yogurt or dairy-free yogurt
1 cup mixed blackberries, raspberries, and blueberries
1 teaspoon ground flaxseeds
2 tablespoons granola, or ¼ cup whole-grain cereal, for crunch (optional)
1 teaspoon unsweetened coconut flakes

▶ *English muffin with cashew butter and berries*

1 whole-grain English muffin, or 2 rye crisps, or 2 rice cakes
1 tablespoon cashew butter or your favorite nut butter
1 cup blueberries, or ½ grapefruit

▶ *Veggie omelet with side of strawberries and blackberries*

1 egg, or 2–3 egg whites, or ⅓ cup egg substitute
Chopped mixed vegetables—broccoli, cauliflower, spinach, red peppers
Fresh basil, chopped
Olive oil to coat pan

(Try making this in an oversized mug!)

1 cup strawberries and blackberries

Brunch

▶ *Whole-grain farina with blueberries and toasted almonds*

1 cup fat-free or low-fat milk or unsweetened milk swap
¼ cup whole-grain farina
¾ cup blueberries (cooked with the farina)
2 tablespoons toasted almonds
Cinnamon and vanilla to taste

▶ *Smoked salmon avocado toast*

Sprouted whole-grain English muffin
¼ medium avocado, mashed
2 ounces smoked salmon
½ heirloom tomato, sliced

▶ *Vegetable frittata*

2 eggs, or 4–6 egg whites, or ½ cup egg substitute
1 cup cut-up raw spinach
½ cup chopped red and yellow bell peppers
½ cup chopped cherry tomatoes
1 tablespoon chopped scallions
1 tablespoon Parmesan cheese
1 slice sprouted whole-grain toast, rye toast, or whole-wheat toast with
    2 tablespoons smashed avocado (optional)

❥ *Peanut butter banana pancakes with berries*

1 whole-grain waffle or pancake (about 4 inches in diameter)
½ cup berries
½ cup fresh banana
2 teaspoons peanut butter, or 4 ounces low-fat Greek yogurt

❥ *Kale and butternut squash frittata*

2 eggs, or 4–6 egg whites, or tofu scramble (3 ounces)
1 cup kale
1 cup roasted butternut squash
Olive oil to coat pan
Herbs and spices as desired

❥ *Warm barley cereal with berry compote*

¼ cup barley
1 cup water (to boil the barley)
¼ cup low-fat milk, almond milk, or your favorite milk swap
1 cup raspberries and blueberries, simmered until compote forms

❥ *Poached eggs with asparagus and tomatoes*

2 eggs, poached
5–6 asparagus spears, sautéed
½ cup cherry tomatoes, sautéed

❥ *Overnight oats with blackberries, pear, and walnuts*

¾ cup fat-free milk, low-fat milk, or your favorite unsweetened nut milk
½ cup old-fashioned or quick whole-grain oats, dry
½ sliced pear
½ cup blackberries
Cinnamon
Vanilla extract to taste
1 tablespoon chopped walnuts

(Mix the ingredients in a mason jar or place them in a bowl, cover, and soak overnight. Heat and eat the next day.)

Lunch and Dinner Options

You can choose to begin dinner with a bowl of vegetable soup, 8–10 ounces. Unless your entrée is a salad, you can start with a mixed salad composed of your favorite vegetables and topped with 1 table-spoon salad dressing or olive oil (and unlimited lemon and vinegar).

❯ Grilled salmon with kasha and rainbow carrots

4–6 ounces salmon, grilled
½ cup kasha, cooked
1 cup rainbow carrots, baked
1–2 teaspoons olive oil

❯ Riced cauliflower with chicken and veggies

1 cup riced cauliflower
1 cup mixed veggies (snap peas, carrots, broccoli, onions) sautéed in olive oil
4 ounces grilled chicken
2 teaspoons low-sodium soy sauce or teriyaki sauce (optional)

❯ Open-faced veggie or tuna burger with avocado and side of green beans

½ whole-grain kaiser roll or sprouted whole-grain English muffin
1 veggie burger or tuna burger
2 tablespoons mashed avocado
1 cup steamed green beans, or 1 cup spaghetti squash topped with fresh tomatoes

❯ Lentil salad with side of hummus, pita, and carrots

½ cup lentils over endive, radicchio, and watercress salad with chopped
    peppers and cucumbers
2 teaspoons olive oil, 1 teaspoon balsamic vinegar, and a squeeze of fresh
    lemon (dressing for lentil salad)
¼ cup hummus and 1 whole-wheat pita (1 ounce)
1 cup cooked carrots with 1 teaspoon olive oil

❯ Open-faced turkey sandwich with arugula and apple

1 slice whole-grain bread, or small pita (1 ounce), or 7-inch tortilla
3 ounces sliced turkey
2 teaspoons Dijon mustard
½ cup arugula
½ sliced apple

*(You have the option to go breadless and add a mixed vegetable salad with 1
    tablespoon balsamic vinaigrette.)*

▶ *Lemon-poached bass with beet-quinoa salad*

4 ounces striped bass
½ lemon, sliced
Olive oil drizzle and spices
1 cup cooked quinoa or kasha
1 cup roasted beets

▶ *Stir-fry with tempeh (or tofu or chicken) and veggies*

1 cup brown rice
1½ cups mixed vegetables (broccoli, bell peppers, snap peas)
3 ounces tempeh, tofu, or white-meat chicken, cubed
1 tablespoon sesame oil
1 tablespoon low-sodium soy sauce

▶ *Black bean burger with pineapple salsa*

1 black bean burger
1 baked potato drizzled with olive oil, or 1 whole-grain roll
2 tablespoons pineapple salsa
1 cup roasted eggplant

▶ *Mediterranean fish*

5–6 ounces flounder, filet of sole, or red snapper broiled with lemon, parsley, spices, and a drizzle of olive oil
1½ cups broccoli slaw or mixed vegetables seasoned with 2 teaspoons olive oil, fresh garlic, lemon, and spices
½ cup whole-grain couscous or brown rice

(Try some grilled artichoke to start.)

▶ *Butternut squash soup with barley and walnut salad*

1 bowl (10 ounces) butternut squash soup
½ cup cooked barley
2 tablespoons chopped walnuts
1 ounce feta cheese
2 cups mixed greens
2–3 teaspoons olive oil, vinegar, and fresh lemon

▶ *Zoodles (zucchini noodles) with chicken and white beans*

3 ounces chicken breast
½ cup white beans
1 medium zucchini, spiraled
1 tablespoon sesame oil
1 cup mixed sautéed vegetables (such as onion, mushrooms, peppers)

▶ *Salmon, tofu, or chicken teriyaki*

4–5 ounces salmon, tofu, or chicken
1 cup cooked mixed vegetables of choice
1 cup cooked brown rice or wild rice
Teriyaki sauce

▶ *Stuffed acorn squash with quinoa, goat cheese (or white beans), and figs*

1 small acorn squash, split in half, roasted
½ cup cooked quinoa
⅓ cup goat cheese, or ½ cup white beans
2 tablespoons chopped dried figs

▶ *Sesame salmon (or your favorite fish) with bok choy and snap peas*

4 ounces salmon, baked
1 tablespoon low-sodium soy sauce
1 cup bok choy, steamed
1 cup snap peas, steamed
1 teaspoon sesame seeds for sprinkling
1 tablespoon sesame oil for drizzling

▶ *Black bean–sweet potato chili*

½ cup black beans
½ medium sweet potato or baked potato, chopped
¼ cup chopped onion
½ cup chopped bell peppers
¾ cup canned diced tomatoes
Olive oil and garlic to taste

❱ *Veggie and hummus pita with side salad*

1 whole-wheat pita (1 ounce)
¼ cup red pepper hummus
½ cup chickpeas
¼ cup tahini
1 cup mixed sautéed vegetables (such as eggplant, red peppers, and zucchini)
1½ cups mixed greens

❱ *Grilled chicken, roasted butternut squash, and onion kebabs*

4 ounces chicken breast
1 cup roasted butternut squash
½ small onion, sliced
1 cup tomato-cucumber salad
1 tablespoon lemon juice
1 teaspoon olive oil

❱ *Spaghetti squash with oodles of vegetables*

2–3 cups spaghetti squash
Broccoli, cauliflower, eggplant, and carrots, sautéed with 1 tablespoon olive oil
   and garlic, topped with 1 cup fresh tomato sauce, 1 ounce shredded part-
   skim mozzarella cheese, 2 tablespoons Parmesan cheese, and fresh garlic,
   spices, and fresh herbs to taste

(For a dairy-free option, substitute ½ cup cooked white beans for the cheeses.)

❱ *Skirt steak or grilled tempeh with sweet potato–kale salad*

4 ounces grilled tempeh or skirt steak
½ cup roasted sweet potatoes
1½ cups kale salad
1 tablespoon dried cranberries
1 tablespoon olive oil

❱ *Tuna Niçoise salad*

1½ cups arugula
3 ounces tuna
½ cup cherry tomatoes
3 small new potatoes, sliced
1 tablespoon lemon or balsamic vinaigrette
5–6 olives

▶ *Asian peanut noodles with veggies*

1½ cups soba noodles
1 tablespoon smooth all-natural peanut butter
1 tablespoon low-sodium soy sauce
1 cup mixed vegetables (mushrooms, peppers, cauliflower, broccoli)
1 teaspoon grated ginger

▶ *Veggie pizza*

1 slice whole-wheat or gluten-free vegetable pizza, topped with spinach,
    onions, broccoli, and eggplant, part-skim mozzarella cheese, and marinara
    sauce, and sprinkled with 1 teaspoon Parmesan cheese, pepper, and
    oregano

▶ *Kale Caesar salad*

1–2 cups chopped kale and shaved Brussels sprouts, with 2 teaspoons Caesar
    dressing
Top with protein of choice: 3 ounces chicken or fish or 1 cup beans or lentils

▶ *Southwest chicken salad with gazpacho*

3–4 ounces grilled chicken
¼ cup corn
¼ cup black beans
½ cup cherry tomatoes
2 cups spinach
Lime dressing (1 tablespoon lime juice, 1 teaspoon olive oil)
1 cup gazpacho

▶ *Baked cod with roasted vegetables*

4–5 ounces baked cod
½ cup Brussels sprouts, roasted
½ cup cauliflower, roasted
½ cup beets, roasted
1 tablespoon olive oil (for roasting)
1 tablespoon chopped fresh sage
1 tablespoon chopped fresh thyme

▶ *Pasta primavera*

1½ cups pasta (whole-wheat pasta, chickpea pasta, or soba noodles)
Sautéed mixed vegetables as desired (cauliflower, broccoli, carrots, spinach,
    zucchini, eggplant)
2–3 teaspoons olive oil
½–¾ cup fresh tomato or marinara sauce
2–3 tablespoons Parmesan cheese (optional)

▶ *Grilled chicken with Brussels sprouts and broccoli and wild rice*

2 cups roasted Brussels sprouts and broccoli
1 tablespoon olive oil and garlic
4 ounces grilled chicken breast
½ cup cooked wild rice blend or quinoa

▶ *Edamame, chickpea, and walnut salad*

2 cups mesclun
½ cup chickpeas
½ cup edamame
¼ cup walnuts, toasted
1 tablespoon balsamic vinaigrette dressing

▶ *Spinach zucchini lasagna*

1 zucchini, sliced
1 cup spinach
½ cup tomato sauce
¼ cup part-skim ricotta cheese
3 tablespoons shredded part-skim mozzarella cheese

*(Cook the vegetables first. Then, in a microwave-safe dish or baking dish, layer
    the vegetables, cheese, and sauce. Bake or microwave.)*

▶ *Veggie burger with soup, salad, and baked potato*

1 cup split pea soup
1 veggie burger
1½ cups mixed greens
Tomato, cucumber, and fresh parsley
2 teaspoons balsamic vinaigrette
1 medium baked potato drizzled with olive oil and sprinkled with Parmesan
    cheese

Snack Options

▶ *Berry parfait*
1 plain or vanilla low-fat Greek yogurt (6–8 ounces)
1 cup berries

▶ *1 medium apple (Fuji, Honeycrisp) with 1 tablespoon almond, peanut, or cashew butter*

▶ *¼ cup black bean dip with 1 cup baby carrots and sliced bell peppers*

▶ *1 pear with ¼ cup pumpkin seeds or almonds*

▶ *Hummus with veggie sticks*
Red pepper, jicama, and celery sticks
½ cup hummus

▶ *Veggies and avocado*
¼ avocado
1 teaspoon chopped onion, ½ cup chopped peppers, and ¼ cup chopped
    tomatoes
1 teaspoon lime juice
Red pepper flakes
1 ounce whole-grain crackers (Mary's Gone Crackers, Kavli, Ryvita, Wasa) or
    large brown rice cake (Lundberg Family Farms) (optional)

▶ *Baked apple drizzled with cinnamon, vanilla, nutmeg, and walnuts*

▶ *Goat cheese zucchini boats*
1 medium zucchini, sliced in half
2 tablespoons goat cheese, or ⅓ cup white beans
1 cup kale, sautéed
4 cherry tomatoes, chopped

❯ South-of-the-border mushroom

1 large portobello mushroom
¼ cup black beans
¼ cup corn
2 tablespoons salsa

❯ Roasted turnips with thyme

1 medium turnip, sliced
1 tablespoon fresh thyme, chopped
1 teaspoon olive oil
Salt and pepper to taste

❯ Cumin-spiced carrots

4 large carrots, peeled and sliced into strips
1 teaspoon olive oil
¼ teaspoon cumin

❯ Poached pear with Greek yogurt or almond yogurt

1 pear, poached
½ cup plain or vanilla low-fat Greek yogurt, or almond yogurt, or 2 teaspoons
  nut butter

❯ Broccoli slaw with water chestnuts, scallions, red peppers, and slivered almonds in a sesame dressing

❯ Israeli salad, 1 cup

Mixed cucumbers and tomato, diced
1 teaspoon olive oil
Fresh lemon juice and fresh chopped parsley to taste

❯ Caprese skewers

1 ounce part-skim mozzarella cheese, cut into small pieces
1 cup cherry tomatoes
Fresh basil
1 teaspoon balsamic glaze

❯ Mini mushroom pizzas

6 button mushrooms
¼ cup chopped cherry tomatoes
1 ounce mozzarella cheese
Dried oregano and basil

Fun yet Healthy Snacks

❯ Chocolate–peanut butter strawberries

6 strawberries
1 tablespoon peanut butter
1 tablespoon cacao nibs

❯ Baked fruit

Fruit of choice—chopped apple, pear, and, plum

*(Cut up the fruit, drizzle on olive oil, add water, and bake in oven. Mix 2 fruits to
make a batch for two days.)*

½ cup frozen yogurt (optional)

❯ Peanut butter–apple pizzas

2 graham cracker squares
2 teaspoons peanut butter
½ sliced apple, or 2 teaspoons dried cherries

❯ Cheesy popcorn

3 cups air-popped popcorn
2 tablespoons Parmesan cheese, or 1 ounce part-skim mozzarella cheese stick

❯ Chocolate-banana frozen yogurt bites

1 banana, sliced
½ cup low-fat vanilla Greek yogurt
1 tablespoon cocoa chips

(Freeze for 1 hour.)

▶ *Apple pie in a mug*

Chopped apple

2 teaspoons chopped walnuts

Cinnamon, vanilla, nutmeg, and a drizzle of lemon juice

(Mix together and bake in a mug.)

▶ *Raspberry-banana "nice cream"*

1 frozen banana

½ cup raspberries

½ cup plain low-fat yogurt

½ cup almond or cashew milk, fat-free milk, or low-fat milk

1 tablespoon toasted almond slivers, or 2 teaspoons hemp heart toppers
    (coconut and cocoa flavor) for topping

Store-Bought: Healthy Grab 'n' Go Portioned Snacks

▶ **Freeze-dried fruit,** small bag (1 ounce)—apple, pineapple, cantaloupe, mango (Crispy Green, Brothers All Natural)

▶ **Roasted chickpeas or edamame,** ¼ cup or 1 ounce (Gold Emblem Abound)

▶ **Freeze-dried vegetables,** 1 ounce—carrots, corn, peas, bell peppers, tomatoes (Just Veggies)

▶ **Beet chips or kale chips,** small bag (1 ounce) (Rhythm Superfoods)

▶ **Ancient grain crisps,** small bag (1 ounce) (Nourish Snacks)

▶ **Mini nut bar** (KIND minis) or 1 small package fruit bites (KIND)

▶ **Bean crisps,** small bag (1 ounce) (Enlightened Roasted Broad Bean Crisps)

Bonus Bites

To save time, use these preportioned single-serve nut and seed packs in the snack recipes.

▶ **Almonds,** 100-calorie pack (Blue Diamond)

▶ **Almond butter,** single-serve squeeze pouch (Justin's)

▶ **Flaxseeds,** single-serve Flax Paks (Carrington Farms)

▶ **Peanut butter,** single-serve squeeze pouch (Crazy Richard's)

▶ **Pistachios,** 100-calorie pack, raw, unsalted (Wonderful)

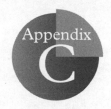

Appendix
C

Portion Tracker

Using the Portion Tracker is easy:

1. Write down what you eat and drink throughout the day, including your portion size and method of preparation.
2. Indicate the correct food group and number of servings for each entry.
3. Cross off each food group serving (with an X) on the diary corresponding to the correct food group icon. If you ate half a serving, cross off with a slash (/).
4. Check to see that you ate the correct number of servings from each food group to match your plan.
5. Be sure to track water, exercise, daily progress, and daily gratitude.

Food (include method of preparation)	Your portion	Food group	Number of servings
BREAKFAST:			
LUNCH:			
SNACK:			
DINNER:			
TREAT (OPTIONAL):			
SNACK:			

Vegetables (Non-starchy)	Fruits	Starches (Grains & Starchy Vegetables)	Fish, Poultry, Meat, & Meat Alternatives	Dairy	Fats

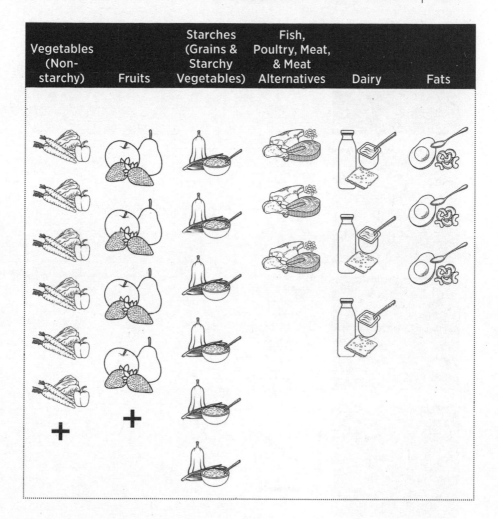

Treats & Sweets:

Water:

Exercise:

Daily Progress:

Daily Gratitude:

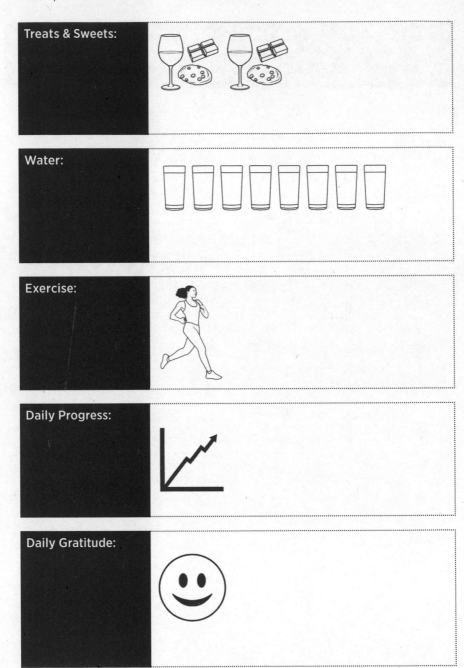

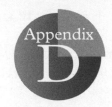

Portion Props

Consider these and other portion props to help you portion control, carry, and store your favorite foods.

Measuring Cups and Spoons

Livliga LivSpoons serving spoons

Leepiya collapsible measuring spoons and cups

OXO Good Grips three-piece angled liquid measuring cup set

Pyrex 3-piece glass measuring cup set (for liquids)

Simply Gourmet stainless steel measuring cups and measuring
  spoons set

Scales

EatSmart digital nutrition scale

Greater Goods Nourish digital kitchen food scale

Plates, Bowls, Glasses, and Mugs

Livliga Celebrate sixteen-piece portion control dinnerware set

Livliga Just Right set

Meal Measure portion control plate

Precise Portions three-piece set: porcelain plate, bowl, and
  drinking glass

Wine-Trax portion control wineglasses

Uno Casa portion control serving bowls

Spray Bottles

Evo oil sprayer bottle

Misto aluminum olive oil sprayer

Prepara oil mister

Food Containers for Meal Prep and Storage

Bento box

Mason jar

Glass food-storage containers

Plastic food-storage and travel containers

Portion Perfection Snacker

Thermos Stainless King 16-ounce food jar with folding
spoon

Cooking Tools, Blenders, Spiralizers

Oster BLSTPB-WBL My Blend blender with travel sport
bottle

Delightly spaghetti measure tool

Jokari pasta portion control containers

Ninja Intelli-Sense kitchen system with auto spiralizer

Perfect Slice square cake pan

Salbree microwave popcorn popper, silicone popcorn maker

Spiralizer five-blade vegetable slicer and veggie pasta and
spaghetti maker

Water Bottles

Great Gear infuser water bottle

Nalgene Tritan water bottle

OMorc sport fruit infuser water bottle

S'well stainless steel water bottle

Thermos Intak hydration bottle

Common Portion Equivalents

Liquid to Volume Conversions

1 fluid ounce = 2 tablespoons
2 fluid ounces = ¼ cup = 4 tablespoons
4 fluid ounces = ½ cup = 8 tablespoons
8 fluid ounces = 1 cup = 16 tablespoons
16 fluid ounces = 2 cups = 1 pint
32 fluid ounces = 4 cups = 1 quart
64 fluid ounces = 8 cups = 2 quarts = ½ gallon
128 fluid ounces = 16 cups = 4 quarts = 1 gallon

US to Metric Conversions

Weight Measures

1 ounce = 28 grams (slightly rounded)
4 ounces = 112 grams = ¼ pound
8 ounces = 224 grams = ½ pound
16 ounces = 448 grams = 1 pound

Liquid Measures

1 teaspoon = 5 milliliters

1 tablespoon = 15 milliliters

1 fluid ounce = 30 milliliters

4 fluid ounces = 120 milliliters

8 fluid ounces = 240 milliliters

2 cups (1 pint) = 480 milliliters

4 cups (1/quart) = 960 milliliters = .96 liter

33 fluid ounces = 1,000 milliliters = 1 liter

4 quarts (1 gallon) = 3.8 liters

Useful Food Yields

4 ounces uncooked poultry, fish, or beef cooks down to about 3 ounces

8 ounces uncooked poultry, fish, or beef cooks down to about 6 ounces

½ cup uncooked oatmeal = 1 cup cooked

1 ounce uncooked pasta = ½ cup cooked

2 ounces uncooked pasta = 1 cup cooked

8 ounces uncooked pasta = 4 cups cooked

3 tablespoons uncooked rice = ½ cup cooked

1 cup uncooked rice = about 4 cups cooked

Acknowledgments

I am deeply grateful to have dedicated colleagues, family, and friends who offered their support throughout the process of researching and writing this book. *Finally Full, Finally Slim* would not have been possible without them.

A heartfelt thank-you to my literary agent, Linda Konner, for her enthusiasm in this project from the first time we met and for her thoughtful advice and encouragement. My deepest gratitude to Karen Chernyaev, whose writing and editing helped to bring out my best voice possible. A special thanks to Christopher Jiménez for creating wonderful illustrations at record speed.

I felt encouraged by the publishing team at Center Street. I am grateful to my editor, Adrienne Ingrum, and assistant editor, Grace Tweedy Johnson, for their expertise, editorial guidance, and commitment throughout the publishing process. I felt lucky to work with Christina Boys in the early stages of this book. A special thanks to Edward Crawford for the creative cover design.

My sincere appreciation to Marion Nestle, my mentor and colleague at New York University (NYU), for her inspiration and support. A special thank-you to the Department of Nutrition and Food Studies at NYU for giving me the opportunity to teach nutrition for twenty-plus years and to my students for asking great questions that keep me thinking. I am also thankful to the many nutrition professionals and talented researchers for sharing their work and for their wonderful contributions to the emerging field of portion control.

Thank you to the National Center for Chronic Disease Prevention and Health Promotion at the Centers for Disease Control and Prevention for recognizing my work and creating *The New (Ab)Normal* infographic based on my research, the perfect image to emphasize growing portions; I am especially grateful to Amanda Dudley and Rita Brett for their immediate response and for working with our production guidelines. Thanks to Anne Agrocostea, Ximena Diz, Isabela Lanes, and Colleen Topper for diligent research assistance.

I am grateful to my clients and readers, who over the years have shared with me their struggles and successes, which has helped me to develop practical solutions. Their weight-loss journeys have inspired me.

As I wrote in *Finally Full, Finally Slim*, friendship and community are vital to good health. I am so fortunate to have colleagues and friends who provided helpful suggestions and support throughout. I am indebted to Adrienne Forman for reading the manuscript and offering helpful suggestions. A special thanks to Dawn Jackson Blatner, Paula Dietz, and Ellie Krieger for their thoughtful insight and recommendations. I am grateful to Dina Benun, Lauren Finkelstein, Michele Harris, Lori Jacobowitz, Kelly James, Susan Karpel, Karen Miller, Eryn Oberlander, Jessica Rackman, Liz Chibnik Rosenblatt, Eva Stein, and Steve Steinberg for help and support along the way; and to Robyn Barsky, Sharon Garfunkel, Donna Lippman, Sharon Kramer Loew, and the entire women's learning group at KJB for showing me the true value of community.

Finally, my deepest appreciation and gratitude to my wonderful family for their love, unwavering support, and encouragement throughout this process and throughout my entire life. Thank you, Mom and Dad, Bonnie, Luca, Teo, Celia, and Brando. Your unconditional love is forever reassuring.

Notes

Gaining Weight? It's Your Portions!

1 Hollands GJ, Shemilt I, Marteau TM, et al. Portion, package or tableware size for changing selection and consumption of food, alcohol and tobacco. *Cochrane Database Syst Rev.* 2015;9:CD011045. doi:10.1002/14651858.CD 011045.pub2.

2 Robinson E, Kersbergen I. Portion size and later food intake: evidence of the "normalizing" effect of reducing food portion sizes. *Am J Clin Nutr.* 2018;107:640–646. doi:10.1093/ajcn/nqy013.

3 Young LR, Nestle M. Reducing portion sizes to prevent obesity: a call to action. *Am J Prev Med.* 2012;43(5):565–568. doi:10.1016/j.amepre .2012.07.024; Young LR, Nestle M. Expanding portion sizes in the US marketplace: implications for nutrition counseling. *J Am Diet Assoc.* 2003;103:231–234. doi:10.1053/jada.2003.50027; Young LR, Nestle M. The contribution of expanding portion sizes to the US obesity epidemic. *Am J Public Health.* 2002;92(2):246–249.

4 Hales CM, Carroll MD, Fryar CD, Ogden CL. Prevalence of obesity among adults and youth: United States, 2015–2016. *NCHS Data Brief* 288. Hyattsville, MD: National Center for Health Statistics; 2017; Hales CM, Fryar CD, Carroll MD, Freedman DS, Ogden CL. Trends in obesity and severe obesity prevalence in US youth and adults by sex and age, 2007–2008 to 2015–2016. *JAMA.* 2018. doi.org/10.1001/jama.2018.3060.

5 Ford E, Dietz W. Trends in energy intake among adults in the United States: findings from NHANES. *Am J Clin Nutr.* 2013;97(4):848–853. doi:10.3945 /ajcn.112.052662; Food availability (per capita) data system: nutrient availability. US Department of Agriculture Economic Research Service. https:// www.ers.usda.gov/data-products/food-availability-per-capita-data-system/. Updated November 23, 2016. Accessed July 3, 2017.

6 Urban LE, Weber JE, Heyman MB, et al. Energy contents of frequently ordered restaurant meals and comparison with human energy requirements

and US Department of Agriculture database information: a multisite randomized study. *J Acad Nutr Diet.* 2016;116(4):590–598. doi:10.1016/j.jand .2015.11.009.

7   Xtreme Eating 2018. Center for Science in the Public Interest website. https://cspinet.org/xtreme-eating-2018. Published 2018. Accessed July 30, 2018.

8   Young LR. *The Portion Teller Plan: The No-Diet Reality Guide to Eating, Cheating, and Losing Weight Permanently.* New York: Crown Publishing Group; 2005.

9   Davis B, Payne CR, Bui AM. Making small food units seem regular: how larger table size reduces calories to be consumed. *J Assoc Consum Res.* 2016;1(1):115–124. doi:10.1086/684527.

10 Rolls BJ, Roe LS, Meengs JS, et al. Increasing the portion size of a sandwich increases energy intake. *J Am Diet Assoc.* 2004;104:367–372. doi:10.1016/j .jada.2003.12.013.

11 French SA, Mitchell NR, Wolfson J, et al. Portion size effects on weight gain in a free living setting. *Obesity (Silver Spring).* 2014:22:1400–1405. doi:10.1002/oby.20720.

12 Wood CT, Skinner AC, Yin HS, et al. Bottle size and weight gain in formula-fed infants. *Pediatrics.* 2016:138(1). http://pediatrics.aappublications.org /content/138/1/e20154538.

13 Block JP, Condon SK, Kleinman K, et al. Consumers' estimation of calorie content at fast food restaurants: cross sectional observational study. *BMJ.* 2013;346:1–10. doi:10.1136/bmj.f2907.

14 Keenan GS, Childs L, Rogers PJ, Hetherington MM, Brunstrom JM. The portion size effect: women demonstrate an awareness of eating more than intended when served larger than normal portions. *Appetite.* 2018;126:54–60. doi:10.1016/j.appet.2018.03.009.

15 McCann MT, Wallace JMW, Robson PJ, et al. Influence of nutrition labeling on food portion size consumption. *Appetite.* 2013;65;153–158; Faulkner GP, Pourshahidi LK, Wallace JMW, Ker MA, McCaffrey TA, Livingstone MBE. Perceived "healthiness" of foods can influence consumers' estimations of energy density and appropriate portion size. *Int J Obes.* 2014;38(1):106–112. doi:10.1038/ijo.2013.69.

16 Food labeling: revision of the nutrition and supplement facts labels. *Federal Register.* US Food and Drug Administration. https://www.federal register.gov/documents/2016/05/27/2016-11867/food-labeling-revision -of-the-nutrition-and-supplement-facts-labels. Published May 27, 2016. Accessed November 1, 2017; Changes to the nutrition facts label. US Food and Drug Administration. https://www.fda.gov/Food/GuidanceRegula tion/GuidanceDocumentsRegulatoryInformation/LabelingNutrition /ucm385663.htm. Updated November 11, 2017. Accessed January 22, 2018.

The Finally Full, Finally Slim Portion Plan

1 US Department of Agriculture. MyPlate. Washington, DC; 2011. www
.choosemyplate.gov. Accessed February 12, 2018.

2 US Department of Health and Human Services and US Department of Agriculture. *2015–2020 Dietary Guidelines for Americans*. 8th ed. Washington, DC; 2015;47. Available at http://health.gov/dietaryguidelines/2015/guidelines/.

3 US Department of Health and Human Services and US Department of Agriculture. *2015–2020 Dietary Guidelines for Americans*. 8th ed. Washington, DC; 2015;43; Lee-Kwan SH, Moore LV, Blanck HM, et al. Disparities in state-specific adult fruit and vegetable consumption—United States, 2015. *MMWR Morb Mortal Wkly Rep*. 2017;66:1241–1247. doi:10.15585/mmwr.mm6645a1.

4 O'Neil PM, Miller-Kovach K, Tuerk PW, et al. Randomized controlled trial of a nationally available weight control program tailored for adults with type 2 diabetes. *Obesity*. 2016;4:2269–2277. doi:10.1002/oby.21616.

5 Newby P, Maras J, Bakun P, Muller D, Ferrucci L, Tucker KL. Intake of whole grains, refined grains, and cereal fiber measured with 7-d diet records and associations with risk factors for chronic disease. *Am J Clin Nutr*. 2007;86(6):1745–1753.

6 US Department of Health and Human Services and US Department of Agriculture. *2015–2020 Dietary Guidelines for Americans*. 8th ed. Washington, DC; 2015;48.

7 US Department of Health and Human Services and US Department of Agriculture. *2015–2020 Dietary Guidelines for Americans*. 8th ed. Washington, DC; 2015;49.

8 The American Heart Association's diet and lifestyle recommendations. American Heart Association website. http://www.heart.org/HEARTORG/HealthyLiving/HealthyEating/Nutrition/The-American-Heart-Associations-Diet-and-Lifestyle-Recommendations_UCM_305855_Article.jsp#.WqCXbGrwaM8. Accessed February 15, 2018; Widmer AJ, Flammer AJ, Lerman LO, et al. The Mediterranean diet, its components, and cardiovascular disease. *Am J Med*. 2015;128(3):229–238. doi:10.1016/h.amjmed.2014.10.014.

9 US Department of Health and Human Services and US Department of Agriculture. *2015–2020 Dietary Guidelines for Americans*. 8th ed. Washington, DC; 2015;49.

10 US Department of Health and Human Services and US Department of Agriculture. *2015–2020 Dietary Guidelines for Americans*. 8th ed. Washington, DC; 2015;23.

11 Sacks FM, Lichtenstein AH, Wu JH. Dietary fats and cardiovascular disease: a presidential advisory from the American Heart Association. *Circulation*. 2017;135:1–25. doi:10.1161/CIR.0000000000000510.

12 Quealy K, Sanger-Katz M. Is sushi "healthy"? What about granola? Where Americans and nutritionists disagree. *New York Times*. July 5, 2016. https://www.nytimes.com/interactive/2016/07/05/upshot/is-sushi-healthy-what-about-granola-where-americans-and-nutritionists-disagree.html. Accessed October 28, 2017.

13 St-Onge MP, Bosarge A. Weight-loss diet that includes consumption of medium-chain triacylglycerol oil leads to a greater rate of weight and fat mass loss than does olive oil. *Am J Clin Nutr*. 2008;87(3):621–626.

14 Saturated fats: why all the hubbub over coconuts? American Heart Association website. https://news.heart.org/saturated-fats-why-all-the-hubbub-over-coconuts/. Published January 21, 2017. Accessed September 19, 2017; Sacks FM, Lichtenstein AH, Wu JH. Dietary fats and cardiovascular disease: a presidential advisory from the American Heart Association. *Circulation*. 2017;135:1–25. doi:10.1161/CIR.0000000000000510.

15 Mattes RD, Dreher ML. Nuts and healthy body weight maintenance mechanisms. *Asia Pac J Clin Nutr*. 2010;19(1):137–141.

16 Sterling SR, Bertrand B, Judd S, et al. Longitudinal analysis of nut-inclusive diets and body mass index among overweight and obese African American women living in rural Alabama and Mississippi, 2011–2013. *Prev Chronic Dis*. 2012;14(82):1–10. doi:10.5888/pcd14.160595.

Day #1: Adopt a New Attitude

1 Dispenza J. *You Are the Placebo*. Carlsbad, CA: Hay House; 2014:105–122.

2 Hill P, Allemand M, Roberts B. Examining the pathways between gratitude and self-rated physical health across adulthood. *Pers Individ Dif*. 2013;54:92–96. doi:10.1016/j.paid.2012.08.011.

3 Kiernan M, Moore SD, Schoffman DE, et al. Social support for healthy behaviors: scale psychometrics and prediction of weight loss among women in a behavioral program. *Obesity (Silver Spring)*. 2012;20:756–764. doi:10.1038/oby.2011.293.

4 Powell K, Wilcox J, Clonan A, et al. The role of social networks in the development of overweight and obesity among adults: a scoping review. *BMC Public Health*. 2015;15:996–1009. doi:10.1186/s12889-015-2314-0; Christakis NA, Fowler JH. The spread of obesity in a large social network over 32 years. *N Engl J Med*. 2007;357:370–379. doi.org/10.1056/NEJMsa066082; Komaroff A. Social networks can affect weight, happiness. *Harvard Health Blog*. December 16, 2011. https://www.health.harvard.edu/blog/social-networks-can-affect-weight-happiness-201112163983; Accessed February 25, 2018.

5 Hingle M, Wertheim B, Thomson C, et al. Research: optimism and diet quality in the women's health initiative. *J Acad Nutr Diet*. 2014;114:1036–1045. doi:10.1016/j.jand.2013.12.018.

6   Epton T, Harris T, Kane PR, et al. The impact of self-affirmation on health-behavior change: a meta-analysis. *Health Psychol.* 2015;34(3):187–196.

Day #2: Write It before You Bite It

1   Hollis JF, Gullion CM, Stevens VJ, Brantley PJ, Appel LJ, Ard JD, et al. for the Weight Loss Maintenance Trial Research Group (2008). Weight loss during the intensive intervention phase of the weight-loss maintenance trial. *American Journal of Preventive Medicine,* 35(2):118–126. doi:10.1016/j.amepre.2008.04.013.
2   Sciamanna CN, Kiernan M, Rolls BJ, et al. Practices associated with weight loss versus weight-loss maintenance. *Am J Prev Med.* 2011;41(2):159–166. doi:10.1016/j.amepre.2011.04.009.

Day #3: Decode Food Labels

1   Changes to the nutrition facts label. US Food and Drug Administration. https://www.fda.gov/Food/GuidanceRegulation/GuidanceDocumentsReg ulatoryInformation/LabelingNutrition/ucm385663.htm. Updated November 11, 2017. Accessed January 22, 2018.
2   National Health and Nutrition Examination Survey. Centers for Disease Control and Prevention. https://www.cdc.gov/nchs/nhanes/. Updated 2018. Accessed April 1, 2018.
3   Mohr GS, Lichtenstein DR, Janiszewski C. The effect of marketer-suggested serving size on consumer responses: the unintended consequences of consumer attention to calorie information. *J Mark.* 2012;76:59–75.
4   Unrealistic serving sizes understate calories, sodium, saturated fat, says CSPI. Center for Science in the Public Interest. http://cspinet.org/new /201108021.html. Published August 2, 2011. Accessed January 20, 2015.
5   Hydock C, Wilson A, Easwar K. The effects of increased serving sizes on consumption. *Appetite.* 2016;1(10):71–79. doi:10.1016/j.appet.2016.02.156.
6   Dallas SK, Liu PJ, Ubel PA. Potential problems with increasing serving sizes on the nutrition fact label. *Appetite.* 2015;95:577–584. doi:10.1016/j .appet.2015.08.012.
7   Changes to the nutrition facts label. US Food and Drug Administration. https://www.fda.gov/Food/GuidanceRegulation/GuidanceDocumentsReg ulatoryInformation/LabelingNutrition/ucm385663.htm. Updated November 11, 2017. Accessed January 22, 2018.
8   US Department of Health and Human Services and US Department of Agriculture. *2015–2020 Dietary Guidelines for Americans.* 8th ed. Washington, DC; 2015;54.
9   American Heart Association website. http://www.heart.org/HEARTORG /HealthyLiving/HealthyEating/Nutrition/Added-Sugars_UCM_305858 _Article.jsp#.WzPkXtVKiM8. Accessed February 15, 2018.

Day #4: Debunk Health Halos

1   Bernstein JT, Franco-Arellano B, Schermel A, Labonté ME, L'Abbé MR. Healthfulness and nutritional composition of Canadian prepackaged foods with and without sugar claims. *Appl Physiol Nutr Metab.* 2017;42(11):1217–1224. doi:10.1139/apnm-2017-0169.

2   Cleeren K, Geyskens K, Verhoef P, Pennings J. Regular or low-fat? An investigation of the long-run impact of the first low-fat purchase on subsequent purchase volumes and calories. *Int J Res Mark.* 2016;33:896–906. doi:10.1016/j.ijresmar.2016.04.001.

3   Okada EM. Justification effects on consumer choice of hedonic and utilitarian goods. *J Mark Res.* 2005;42(1):43–53. doi:10.1509/jmkr.42.1.43.56889.

4   Calvo-Lerma J, Martínez-Barona S, Crespo-Escobar P, Fornes V, Donat E, Ribes-Koninck C. Comprehensive analysis of the nutritional profile of gluten-free products as compared to their gluten-containing counterparts. Paper presented at the Annual Meeting of the European Society for Pediatric Gastroenterology, Hepatology and Nutrition; May 11, 2017; Prague, Czech Republic. http://www.espghancongress.org/fileadmin/user_upload/Gluten_Free_Products_Press_Release_-_APPROVED.pdf. Accessed November 13, 2017.

5   Schuldt JP, Schwarz N. The "organic" path to obesity? Organic claims influence calorie judgments and exercise recommendations. *Judgm Decis Mak.* 2010;5(3):144–150.

6   Azad MB, Abou-Setta AM, Chauhan BF, et al. Nonnutritive sweeteners and cardiometabolic health: a systematic review and meta-analysis of randomized controlled trials and prospective cohort studies. *Can Med Assoc J.* 2017;189(28):929–939. doi:10.1503/cmaj.161390.

7   Levings J. FDA's new definition of "healthy." *Today's Dietitian.* February 2017. http://www.todaysdietitian.com/newarchives/0217p36.shtml. Accessed February 27, 2017; "Healthy" on food labeling. US Food and Drug Administration (FDA). https://www.fda.gov/food/guidanceregulation/guidancedocumentsregulatoryinformation/labelingnutrition/ucm520695.htm. Published November 11, 2017. Accessed January 18, 2018.

8   Nestle M. Food products with health claims only marginally better (no surprise). FoodPolitics.com website. https://www.foodpolitics.com/2016/08/food-products-with-health-claims-only-marginally-better-no-surprise/. Published August 8, 2016. Accessed March 1, 2018; Nestle M. What does healthy mean on food labels? FoodPolitics.com website. https://www.foodpolitics.com/2016/09/what-does-healthy-mean-on-food-labels/. Published September 26, 2016. Accessed January 25, 2018; Nestle M, Nesheim M. *Why Calories Count: From Science to Politics.* Berkeley: University of California Press; 2013; Nestle M. *Food Politics: How the Food Industry Influences Nutrition and Health.* Revised and expanded 10th anniversary ed. Berkeley: University of California Press; 2013.

9   Whitman IR, Pletcher MJ, Vittinghoff E, et al. Perceptions, information
    sources, and behavior regarding alcohol and heart health. *Am J Cardiol.*
    2015;116(4):642–646. doi:10.1016/j.amjcard.2015.05.029.

Day #5: Eat Food, Not Nutrients

1   Gardner CD, Trepanowski JF, Del Gobbo LC, et al. Effect of low-fat vs
    low-carbohydrate diet on 12-month weight loss in overweight adults and
    the association with genotype pattern or insulin secretion: the DIET-
    FITS randomized clinical trial. *JAMA.* 2018;319(7):667–679. doi:10.1001
    /jama.2018.0245.
2   Stanton MV, Robinson JL, Kirkpatrick SM, et al. DIETFITS study
    (diet intervention examining the factors interacting with treatment suc-
    cess)—study design and methods. *Contemp Clin Trials.* 2017;53:151–161.
    doi:10.1016/j.cct.2016.12.021.
3   Gardner CD, Trepanowski JF, Del Gobbo LC, et al. Effect of low-fat vs
    low-carbohydrate diet on 12-month weight loss in overweight adults and
    the association with genotype pattern or insulin secretion: the DIET-
    FITS randomized clinical trial. *JAMA.* 2018;319(7):667–679. doi:10.1001
    /jama.2018.0245; Stanton MV, Robinson JL, Kirkpatrick SM, et al. DIET-
    FITS study (diet intervention examining the factors interacting with treat-
    ment success)—study design and methods. *Contemp Clin Trials.* 2017;53:
    151–161. doi:10.1016/j.cct.2016.12.021; Dennett C. Low-carb vs. low-fat:
    new research says it doesn't really matter. *Washington Post.* July 17, 2017.
    https://www.washingtonpost.com/lifestyle/wellness/low-carb-vs-low-fat-new
    -research-says-it-doesnt-really-matter/2017/07/13/270d2270-61c1-11e7-a4f7
    -af34fc1d9d39_story. Accessed January 5, 2018.
4   US Department of Health and Human Services and US Department of
    Agriculture. *2015–2020 Dietary Guidelines for Americans.* 8th ed. Washing-
    ton, DC; 2015;15.
5   US Department of Health and Human Services and US Department of
    Agriculture. *2015–2020 Dietary Guidelines for Americans.* 8th ed. Washing-
    ton, DC; 2015;97.
6   Austin GL, Ogden LG, Hill JO. Trends in carbohydrate, fat, and protein
    intakes and association with energy intake in normal-weight, overweight,
    and obese individuals: 1971–2006. *Am J Clin Nutr.* 2011;93(4):836–843.
    doi:10.3945/ajcn.110.000141.
7   Li Y, Hruby A, Bernstein AM, et al. Saturated fats compared with unsatu-
    rated fats and sources of carbohydrates in relation to risk of coronary heart
    disease: a prospective cohort study. *J Am Coll Cardiol.* 2015;66:1538–1548.
    doi:10.1016/j.jacc.2015.07.055.

8   Unrealistic serving sizes understate calories, sodium, saturated fat, says CSPI. Center for Science in the Public Interest website. http://cspinet.org /new/201108021.html. Published August 2, 2011. Accessed January 20, 2015.

Day #6: Get Over Your Fear of Carbs

1   Bentley J. Potatoes and tomatoes account for over half of U.S. vegetable availability. US Department of Agriculture website. September 8, 2015. https:// www.ers.usda.gov/amber-waves/2015/september/potatoes-and-tomatoes -account-for-over-half-of-us-vegetable-availability/. Accessed February 7, 2018.
2   Food availability and consumption. US Department of Agriculture website. https://www.ers.usda.gov/data-products/ag-and-food-statistics-charting -the-essentials/food-availability-and-consumption/. Updated September 14, 2017. Accessed October 14, 2017.
3   US Department of Health and Human Services and US Department of Agriculture. *2015–2020 Dietary Guidelines for Americans*. 8th ed. Washington, DC; 2015:54–55.
4   US Department of Health and Human Services and US Department of Agriculture. *2015–2020 Dietary Guidelines for Americans*. 8th ed. Washington, DC; 2015:48.
5   Newby P, Maras J, Bakun P, Muller D, Ferrucci L, Tucker KL. Intake of whole grains, refined grains, and cereal fiber measured with 7-d diet records and associations with risk factors for chronic disease. *Am J Clin Nutr.* 2007;86(6):1745–1753.
6   Shafique M, Russell S, Murdoch SJ, Bell JD, Guess N. Dietary intake in people consuming a low-carbohydrate diet in the UK Biobank. *J Hum Nutr Diet.* 2018. 31(2):228–238. doi:10.1111/jhn.12527.
7   Boden G, Sargrad K, Homko C, Mozzoli M, Stein T. Effect of a low-carbohydrate diet on appetite, blood glucose levels, and insulin resistance in obese patients with type 2 diabetes. *Ann Intern Med.* 2005;142(6):403–411.
8   Katz DL, Meller S. Can we say what diet is best for health? *Annu Rev Public Health.* 2014;35:83–103. doi:10.1146/annurev-publhealth-032013-182351.

Day #7: Let Your Hand Lead the Way

1   Gibson AA, Hsu MSH, Rangan AM, et al. Accuracy of hands v. household measures as portion size estimation aids. *J Nutr Sci.* 2016;5:1–11. doi:10.1017/jns.2016.22.
2   Flynn MA, O'Brien CM, Faulkner G, Flynn CA, Gajownik M, Burke SJ. Revision of food-based dietary guidelines for Ireland, phase 1: evaluation of Ireland's food guide. *Public Health Nutr.* 2012;15(3):518–526. doi:10.1017 /S1368980011002072.

Day #8: Right-Size Your Dishes

1 Hollands GJ, Shemilt I, Marteau TM, et al. Portion, package or tableware size for changing selection and consumption of food, alcohol and tobacco. *Cochrane Database Syst Rev.* 2015;(9):CD011045. doi:10.1002/14651858 .CD011045.pub2.

2 Pratt IS, Croager EJ, Rosenberg M. The mathematical relationship between dishware size and portion size. *Appetite.* 2012;58:299–302; Klara R. Table the issue: the elements that make up a tabletop can be very important. But do customers really notice them? *Restaurant Business.* 2004;103(18):14.

3 DiSantis K. Birch L, Davey A, et al. Plate size and children's appetite: effects of larger dishware on self-served portions and intake. *Pediatrics.* 2013;131(5):e1451–e1458. doi:10.1542/peds.2012-2330.

4 Zupan Z, Mphil AE, Couturier DL, Marteau TH. Wine glass capacity in England has increased sevenfold in 300 years. Can downsizing reduce wine consumption? *BMJ.* 2017;359:1–5. doi:10.1136/bmj.j5623.

5 Attwood AS, Scott-Samuel NE, Stothart G, Munafo MR. Glass shape influences consumption rate for alcoholic beverages. *PLoS ONE.* 2012;7(8): e43007. doi:10.1371/journal.pone.0043007.

6 Genschow O, Reutner L, Wanke M. The color red reduces snack food and soft drink intake. *Appetite.* 2012;58(2):699–702. doi:10.1016/j.appet.2011 .12.023.

Day #9: Declutter Your Kitchen

1 Walsh, P. *Lose the Clutter, Lose the Weight.* New York: Rodale Books; 2015.

2 de Oliveira Otto MC, Anderson CAM, Dearborn JL, et al. Dietary diversity: implications for obesity prevention in adult populations: a science advisory from the American Heart Association. *J Am Heart Assoc.* 2018;138:00–00. doi:10.1161./CIR.0000000000000595. Raynor HA, Steeves EA, Hecht J, Fava JL, Wing RR. Limiting variety in non-nutrient dense, energy-dense foods during a lifestyle intervention: a randomized controlled trial. *Am J Clin Nutr.* 2012;95(6):1305–1314. doi:10.3945/ajcn.111.031153.

3 2018 Global wellness trends reports: the wellness kitchen. Global Wellness Summit website. https://www.globalwellnesssummit.com/2018-global-wellness -trends/wellness-kitchen/. Published 2018. Accessed April 21, 2018.

4 Nakata R, Kawai N. The social facilitation of eating without the presence of others: self-reflection on eating makes food taste better and people eat more. *Physiol Behav.* 2017;179:23–29. doi:10.1016/j.physbeh.2017.05.022.

Day #10: Cook Like a Portion Pro

1 Wolfson JA, Bleich SN. Is cooking at home associated with better diet quality or weight-loss intention? *Public Health Nutr.* 2014;18(8):1397–1406. doi:10.1017/S1368980014001943.
2 Mills S, Brown H, Wrieden W, White M, Adams J. Frequency of eating home cooked meals and potential benefits for diet and health: cross-sectional analysis of a population-based cohort study. *Int J Behav Nutr Phys Act.* 2017;14:109. doi:10.1186/s12966-017-0567-y; Tiwari A, Aggarwal A, Tang W, Drewnowski A. Cooking at home: a strategy to comply with U.S. Dietary Guidelines at no extra cost. *Am J Prev Med.* 2017;52(5):616–624. doi:10.1016/j.amepre.2017.01.017.
3 Almiron-Roig E, Dominguez A, Vaughan D, et al. Acceptability and potential effectiveness of commercial portion control tools amongst people with obesity. *Br J Nutr.* 2016;116(11):1974–1983. doi:10.1017/S0007114516004104.
4 Leung Lam MC, Adams J. Association between home food preparation skills and behaviour, and consumption of ultra-processed foods: cross-sectional analysis of the UK national diet and nutrition survey (2008–2009). *Int J Behav Nutr Phys Act.* 2017;14:68. doi:10.1186/s12966-017-0524-9.

Day #11: Prepare the Perfect Plate

1 Flood J, Rolls B. Soup preloads in a variety of forms reduce meal energy intake. *Appetite.* 2007;49(3):626–634. doi:10.1016/j.appet.2007.04.002.

Day #12: Think "Whole-istically"

1 Monteiro CA, Cannon G, Moubarac JC, et al. Household availability of ultra-processed foods and obesity in nineteen European countries. *Public Health Nutr.* 2018:21(1):5–17. doi:10.1017/S1368980017001379.
2 AICR Health Talk. American Institute for Cancer Research website. http://www.aicr.org/press/health-features/health-talk/2013/08aug2013/minimally-processed-food.html. Published August 12, 2013. Accessed April 21, 2018.
3 Monteiro CA, Moubarac JC, Bertazzi Levu R, Silva Canella DS, Da Costa Louzada ML, Cannon G. Household availability of ultra-processed foods and obesity in nineteen European countries. *Public Health Nutr.* 2018;21(1):18–26. doi:10.1017/S1368980017001379.
4 AICR Health Talk. American Institute for Cancer Research website. http://www.aicr.org/press/health-features/health-talk/2013/08aug2013/minimally-processed-food.html. Published August 12, 2013. Accessed April 21, 2018.

5   What is processed food? Michigan State University extension website. http://
    msue.anr.msu.edu/news/what_is_a_processed_food. Published November
    26, 2014. Accessed April 21, 2018.
6   Pollan M. *Food Rules: An Eater's Manual.* New York: Penguin Books; 2009.
7   Final determination regarding partially hydrogenated oils (removing
    trans fat). US Food and Drug Administration. https://www.fda.gov/Food
    /IngredientsPackagingLabeling/FoodAdditivesIngredients/ucm449162
    .htm. Published February 27, 2018. Accessed April 21, 2018; Trans fat is
    double trouble for your heart health. Mayo Clinic website. https://www
    .mayoclinic.org/diseases-conditions/high-blood-cholesterol/in-depth/trans
    -fat/art-20046114. Published March 1, 2017. Accessed April 21, 2018.
8   US Department of Health and Human Services and US Department of
    Agriculture. *2015–2020 Dietary Guidelines for Americans.* 8th ed. Washing-
    ton, DC; 2015;34.
9   Jackson SL, King SMC, Zhao L, et al. Prevalence of excess sodium intake in
    the United States—NHANES, 2009–2012. *MMWR Morb Mortal Wkly Rep.*
    64(52);1393–1397.
10 Cut down on sodium. Dietary Guidelines for Americans 2015–2020, 8th ed.
    https://health.gov/dietaryguidelines/2015/resources/DGA_Cut-Down-On
    -Sodium.pdf. Published December 2016. Accessed April 21, 2018; You may
    be surprised by how much salt you're eating. US Food and Drug Adminis-
    tration. https://www.fda.gov/ForConsumers/ConsumerUpdates/ucm327369
    .htm. Published July 19, 2016. Accessed April 21, 2018.
11 Nestle M. *Food Politics: How the Food Industry Influences Nutrition and Health.*
    10th anniversary ed. Oakland: University of California Press; 2013.
12 Qiang L, Yuanting C, Rongbing J, et al. Enjoyment of spicy flavor enhances
    central salty-taste perception and reduces salt intake and blood pressure. *J
    Hypertens.* 2017;70:1291–1299. doi:10.1161/hypertensionaha.117.09950.
13 EWG's 2018 shopper's guide to pesticides in produce. The Environmental
    Working Group. https://www.ewg.org/foodnews/. Published 2018. Accessed
    January 30, 2018.
14 Sotos-Prieto M, Bhupathiraju S, Mattei J, et al. Association of changes in diet
    quality with total and cause-specific mortality. *N Engl J Med.* 2017;377:143–
    153. doi:10.1056/NEJMoa1613502.

Day #13: Fill Up on Freebies

1   Zuraikat FM, Roe LS, Sanchez CE, Rolls BJ. Comparing the portion size
    effect in women with and without extended training in portion control: a
    follow-up to the portion-control strategies trial. *Appetite.* 2018;123:334–342.
    doi:10.1016/j.appet.2018.01.012.

2 Conner TS, Brookie KL, Carr AC, Mainvil LA, Vissers MCM. Let them eat fruit! The effect of fruit and vegetable consumption on psychological well-being in young adults: a randomized controlled trial. *PLoS ONE.* 2017;12(2): e0171206. doi:10.1371/journal.pone.0171206.

3 Roe LS, Meengs JS, Rolls BJ. Salad and satiety: the effect of timing of salad consumption on meal energy intake. *Appetite.* 2012;58(1):242–248. doi:10.1016/j.appet.2011.10.003.

4 David ME, Haws KL. Saying "no" to cake or "yes" to kale: approach and avoidance strategies in pursuit of health goals. *Psychol Mark.* 2016;33(8):588–594. doi:10.1002/mar.2090.

5 Mann T. *Secrets From the Eating Lab.* New York: HarperCollins; 2015.

6 Bouzari A, Holstege D, Barrett DM. Vitamin retention in eight fruits and vegetables: a comparison of refrigerated and frozen storage. *J Agric Food Chem.* 2015;63(3):957–962. doi:10.1021/jf5058793.

7 Rock CL, Flatt SW, Pakiz B, Barkai HS, Heath DD, Krumhar KC. Randomized clinical trial of portion-controlled prepackaged foods to promote weight loss. *Obesity (Silver Spring).* 2016;24:1230–1237. doi:10.1002/oby.21481.

8 Blatt AD, Roe LS, Rolls BJ. Hidden vegetables: an effective strategy to reduce energy intake and increase vegetable intake in adults. *Am J Clin Nutr.* 2011:93(4):756–763. doi:10.3945/ajcn.110.009332.

9 Chernev A. The dieter's paradox. *J Consum Psychol.* 2011;21(2):178–183. doi:10.1016/j.jcps.2010.08.002.

Day #14: Shop Like a Chef

1 Haire C, Raynor HA. Weight status moderates the relationship between package size and food intake. *J Acad Nutr Diet.* 2014;114(8):1251–1256. doi:10.1016/j.jand.2013.12.022.

2 U.S. Food Waste Challenge FAQs. US Department of Agriculture. https://www.usda.gov/oce/foodwaste/faqs.htm. Updated 2018. Accessed February 19, 2018.

3 Frank AP, Clegg DJ. Dietary guidelines for Americans—eat less sugar. *JAMA.* 2016;315(11):1196. doi:10.1001/jama.2016.0968.

4 Georgina Russell C, Burke PF, Waller DS, et al. The impact of front-of-pack marketing attributes versus nutrition and health information on parents' food choices. *Appetite.* 2017;116:323–338. doi.org/10.1016/j.appet.2017.05.001.

5 Lahnakoski JM, Jääskeläinen IP, Sams M, et al. Neural mechanisms for integrating consecutive and interleaved natural events. *Hum Brain Mapp.* 2017;38(7):3360–3376. doi:10.1002/hbm.23591.

6 Aerts G, Smits T. The package size effect: how package size affects young children's consumption of snacks differing in sweetness. *Food Qual Prefer.* 2017;60:72–80. doi:10.1016/j.foodqual.2017.03.015.

7   Women could lose 4.1 lbs simply by avoiding impulse items at the checkout, says new study from IHL Consulting Group. Business Wire website. http://www .businesswire.com/news/home/20070906005261/en/Women-Lose-4.1-lbs -Simply-Avoiding-Impulse. Published September 6, 2007. Accessed April 29, 2017.

8   Chandon P, Ordabayeva N. The accuracy of less: natural bounds explain why quantity decreases are estimated more accurately than quantity increases. *J Exp Psychol*. 2017;146(2):250–268. doi:10.1037/xge0000259.

Day #15: Dine Out Defensively

1   Food prices and spending. US Department of Agriculture website. https:// www.ers.usda.gov/data-products/ag-and-food-statistics-charting-the -essentials/food-prices-and-spending/. Published March 13, 2018. Accessed March 18, 2018.

2   Urban LE, Weber JE, Heyman MB, et al. Energy contents of frequently ordered restaurant meals and comparison with human energy requirements and US Department of Agriculture database information: a multisite randomized study. *J Acad Nutr Diet*. 2016;116(4):590–598. doi:10.1016/jand.2015.11.009.

3   Cohen DA, Lesser LI, Wright C, et al. Kid's menu portion sizes: how much should children be served? *Nutr Today*. 2016;51(6):273–280. doi:10.1097 /NT.0000000000000179.

4   Turnwald BP, Boles DZ, Crum AJ. Association between indulgent descriptions and vegetable consumption: twisted carrots and dynamite beets. *JAMA Intern Med*. 2017;177(8):1216–1218. doi:10.1001/jamainternmed.2017.1637.

5   FDA agrees to enforce menu labeling rule in May 2018. National Consumer League website. http://www.nclnet.org/fda_menu_labeling_rule. Published September 2017. Accessed April 21, 2018.

6   Berkowitz S, Marquart L, Mykerezi E, Degeneffe D, Reicks M. Reduced-portion entrées in a worksite and restaurant setting: impact on food consumption and waste. *Public Health Nutr*. 2016;19(16):3048–3054. doi:10.1017 /S1368980016001348.

7   Schwartz J, Riis J, Elbel B, Ariely D. Inviting consumers to downsize fast-food portions significantly reduces calorie consumption. *Health Aff (Millwood)*. 2012;31(2):399–407. doi:10.1377/hlthaff.2011.0224.

8   An R, Andrade F, Grigsby-Toussaint D. Sandwich consumption in relation to daily dietary intake and diet quality among US adults, 2003–2012. *Public Health*. 2016;140:206–212. doi:10.1016/j.puhe.2016.06.008.

Day #16: Be Your Own General

1   Ducrot P, Méjean C, Péneau S, et al. Meal planning is associated with food variety, diet quality and body weight status in a large sample of French adults. *Int J Behav Nutr Phys Act*. 2017;14:1–12. doi:10.1186/s12966-017-0461-7; Monsivais P, Aggarwai A, Drewnowski A. Time spent on home food preparation and indicators of healthy eating. *Am J Prev Med*. 2014;47(6):796–802. doi:10.1016/j.amepre.2014.07.033.

2   Zimmerman A, Mason A, Rogers PJ, Brunstrom JM. Obese and overweight individuals are less sensitive to information about meal times in portion size judgements. *Int J Obes*. 2017. doi:10.1038/ijo.2017.275.

3   Stroebele-Benschop N, Dieze A, Hilzendegen C. First come, first served. Does pouring sequence matter for consumption? *Appetite*. 2016;105:731–736. doi:10.1016/j.appet.2016.07.011.

4   Rubin G. *Better Than Before*. New York: Broadway Books; 2015.

5   Kliewer KL, Ke JY, Lee HY, et al. Short-term food restriction followed by controlled refeeding promotes gorging behavior, enhances fat deposition, and diminishes insulin sensitivity in mice. *J Nutr Biochem*. 2015;26:721–728. doi:10.1016/j.nutbio.2015.01.010.

Day #17: Eat Mindfully

1   Dalen J, Smith BW, Shelley BM, Sloan AL, Leahigh L, Begay D. Pilot study: mindful eating and living (MEAL): weight, eating behavior, and psychological outcomes associated with a mindfulness-based intervention for people with obesity. *Complement Ther Med*. 2010;18(6):260–264. doi:10.1016/j.ctim.2010.09.008.

2   Niemeier H, Leahey T, Palm Reed K, Brown RA, Wing RR. An acceptance-based behavioral intervention for weight loss: a pilot study. *Behav Ther*. 2012;43(2):427–435. doi:10.1016/j.beth.2011.10.005.

3   Carriere K, Khoury B, Gunak M, Knauper B. Mindfulness-based interventions for weight loss: a systematic review and meta-analysis. *Obes Rev*. 2018;19:164–177. doi:10.1111/obr.12623.

4   Hendrickson K, Rasmussen E. Mindful eating reduces impulsive food choice in adolescents and adults. *Health Psychol*. 2017;36(3):226–235. doi:10.1037/hea0000440.

5   Dunn C, Haubenreiser M, Johnson M, et al. Mindfulness approaches and weight loss, weight maintenance, and weight regain. *Curr Obes Rep*. 2018;7(1):37–49. doi:10.1007/s13679-018-0299-6.

6   Robinson E, Kersbergen I, Higgs S. Eating "attentively" reduces later energy consumption in overweight and obese females. *Br J Nutr*. 2015;112(4):657–661. doi:10.1017/S000711451400141X.

7   Andrade AM, Greene GW, Melanson KJ. Eating slowly led to decreases in energy intake within meals in healthy women. *J Am Diet Assoc.* 2008;108(7): 1186–1191. doi:10.1016/j.jada.2008.04.026.

8   Shah M, Copeland J, Dart L, Adams-Huet B, James A, Rhea D. Slower eating speed lowers energy intake in normal-weight but not overweight/ obese subjects. *J Acad Nutr Diet.* 2014;114(3):393–402. doi:10.1016/j .jand.2013.11.002.

9   Zhu Y, Hollis JH. Increasing the number of chews before swallowing reduces meal size in normal-weight, overweight, and obese adults. *J Acad Nutr Diet.* 2014;114(6):926–931. doi:10.1016/j.jand.2013.08.020.

10 Oldham-Cooper RE, Hardman CA, Nicoll CE, et al. Playing a computer game during lunch affects fullness, memory for lunch, and later snack intake. *Am J Clin Nutr.* 2011;93(2):308–313. doi:10.3945/ajcn.110.004580.

11 Food-based dietary guidelines—Brazil. Food and Agriculture Organization of the United Nations website. http://www.fao.org/nutrition/education /food-based-dietary-guidelines/regions/countries/brazil/en/. Published 2014. Accessed March 1, 2018.

12 Hurst Y, Fukuda H. Effects of changes in eating speed on obesity in patients with diabetes: a secondary analysis of longitudinal health check-up data. *BMJ.* 2018;8:e019589. doi:10.1136/bmjopen-2017-019589.

13 Willcox BJ, Willcox DC, Suzuki M. *The Okinawa Program: How the World's Longest-Lived People Achieve Everlasting Health—and How You Can Too.* New York: Clarkson Potter; 2001.

14 How to know when your stomach is full & when to stop eating? SF Gate website. http://healthyeating.sfgate.com/stomach-full-stop-eating-3080.html. Published March 31, 2018. Accessed April 15, 2018.

Day #18: Swap and Drop

1   Tate DF, Turner-McGrievy G, Lyons E, et al. Replacing caloric beverages with water or diet beverages for weight loss in adults: main results of the Choose Healthy Options Consciously Everyday (CHOICE) randomized clinical trial. *Am J Clin Nutr.* 2012;95(3):555–563. doi:10.3945 /ajcn.111.026278.

2   O'Connor L, Imamura F, Lentjes MAH, et al. Prospective associations and population impact of sweet beverage intake and type 2 diabetes, and effects of substitutions with alternative beverages. *Diabetologia.* 2015;58(7):1474– 1483. doi:10.1007/s00125-015-3572-1.

3   Kristensen M, Toubro S, Jensen MG, et al. Whole grain compared with refined wheat decreases the percentage of body fat following a 12-week, energy-restricted dietary intervention in postmenopausal women. *J Nutr.* 2012;142(4):710–716. doi:10.3945/jn.111.142315.

4   Wrieden W, Levy L. "Change4Life Smart Swaps": quasi-experimental eval-
    uation of a natural experiment. *Public Health Nutr.* 2016;9(13):2388–2392.
    doi:10.1017/S1368980016000513.

5   Calder PC. New evidence that omega-3 fatty acids have a role in primary
    prevention of coronary heart disease. *J Public Health Emerg.* 2017;1(35):1–6.
    doi:10.21037/jphe.2017.03.03.

6   Satija A, Hu FB. Plant-based diets and cardiovascular health. *Trends Cardio-
    vasc Med.* 2018. doi:10.1016/j.tcm.2018.02.004; Malik VS, Tobias DK, Pan
    A, Hu FB. Dietary protein intake and risk of type 2 diabetes in US men and
    women. *Am J Epidemiol.* 2016;183(8):715–728. doi:10.1093/aje/kwv268.

Day #19: Power Up Your Snacks

1   Dunford EK, Popkin BM. Disparities in snacking trends in U.S. adults over
    a 35 year period from 1977–2012. *Nutrients.* 2017;9(8):E809. doi:10.3390
    /nu9080809.

2   As snackification in food culture becomes more routine, traditional meal-
    times get redefined. The Hartman Group website. http://www.hartman
    -group.com/hartbeat/638/as-snackification-in-food-culture-becomes-more
    -routine-traditional-mealtimes-get-redefined. Published February 16, 2016.
    Accessed January 15, 2018.

3   Haire C, Raynor HA. Weight status moderates the relationship between
    package size and food intake. *J Acad Nutr Diet.* 2014;114(8):1251–1256.
    doi:10.1016/j.and.2013.12.022.

4   Ogden J, Wood C, Payne E, Fouracre H, Lammyman F. "Snack" versus
    "meal": the impact of label and place on food intake. *Appetite.* 2018;120(1):666–
    672. doi:10.1016/j.appet.2017.10.026.

5   St-Ogne MP, Ard J, Baskin ML, Chiuve SE, Johnson HM, Kris-Etherton
    P, et al. Meal timing and frequency: implications for cardiovascular disease
    prevention: a scientific statement from the American Heart Association.
    Circulation. 2017;137(16). doi:10.1161/CIR.0000000000000476.

6   Hagen L, Krishna A, McFerran B. Rejecting responsibility: low physical
    involvement in obtaining food promotes unhealthy eating. *J Mark Res.*
    2017;54(4):589–604. doi:10.1509/jmr.14.0125.

Day #20: Sip Your Way to Slim

1   Hu FB. Resolved: there is sufficient scientific evidence that decreasing
    sugar-sweetened beverage consumption will reduce the prevalence of obe-
    sity and obesity-related diseases. *Obes Rev.* 2013;14(8):606–619. doi:10.1111
    /obr.12040; Nestle M. *Soda Politics: Taking on Big Soda (and Winning).* New
    York: Oxford University Press; 2015.

2   Hamada Y, Kashima H, Hayashi N. The number of chews and meal duration affect diet-induced thermogenesis and splanchnic circulation. *Obesity (Silver Spring)*. 2014;22:62–69. doi:10.1002/oby.20715.

3   Chambers L, McCrickerd K, Yeomans MR. Optimising foods for satiety. *Trends Food Sci Technol*. 2015;41(2):149–160. doi:0.1016/j.tifs.2014.10.007.

4   Houchins JA, Tan S, Campbell WW, Mattes RD. Effects of fruit and vegetable, consumed in solid vs. beverage forms, on acute and chronic appetitive responses in lean and obese adults. *Int J Obes (Lond)*. 2013;37(8):1109–1115. doi:10.1038/ijo.2012.183.

5   Young LR. *The Portion Teller Plan: The No-Diet Reality Guide to Eating, Cheating, and Losing Weight Permanently*. New York: Crown; 2005:245–246; Young LR, Nestle M. Reducing portion sizes to prevent obesity: a call to action. *Am J Prev Med*. 2012;43(5):565–568. doi:10.1016/j.amepre.2012.07.024.

6   Bleich SN, Vercammen KA. The negative impact of sugar-sweetened beverages on children's health: an update of the literature. *BMC Obesity*. 2018;5:6. doi:10.1186/s40608-017-0178-9.

7   Ribakove S, Almy J, Wootan MG. Soda on the menu: improvements seen but more change needed for beverages on restaurant children's menus. Center for Science in the Public Interest. https://cspinet.org/sites/default/files/attachment/Soda%20on%20the%20Menu.pdf. Published July 2017. Accessed November 16, 2017.

8   Hu FB. Resolved: there is sufficient scientific evidence that decreasing sugar-sweetened beverage consumption will reduce the prevalence of obesity and obesity-related diseases. *Obes Rev*. 2013;14(8):606–619. doi:10.1111/obr.12040; Stern D, Middaugh N, Rice MS. Changes in sugar-sweetened soda consumption, weight, and waist circumference: 2-year cohort of Mexican women. *J Public Health*. 2017;107:1801–1808. doi:10.2105/AJPH.2017.304008.

9   Feller S. Swapping one sugary drink per day for water has benefit, study says. *UPI*. https://www.upi.com/Health_News/2016/08/15/Swapping-one-sugary-drink-per-day-for-water-has-big-health-benefit-study-says/8661471268957/. Published August 15, 2016. Accessed March 16, 2018; Duffey KJ, Poti J. Modeling the effect of replacing sugar-sweetened beverage consumption with water on energy intake, HBI Score, and obesity prevalence. *Nutrients*. 2016;8(7):395. doi:10.3390/nu8070395.

10 Muraki I, Imamura F, Manson JE, et al. Fruit consumption and risk of type 2 diabetes: results from three prospective longitudinal cohort studies. *BMJ*. 2013;347:f5001. doi:10.1136/bmj.f5001.

11 Deshpande G, Mapanga RF, Faadiel Essop M. Frequent sugar-sweetened beverage consumption and the onset of cardiometabolic diseases: cause for concern? *J Endocr Soc*. 2017;1(11):1372–1385. doi:10.1210/js.2017-00262.

12 Azad M, Ahmed M, Bhupendrasinh C, et al. Nonnutritive sweeteners and cardiometabolic health: a systematic review and meta-analysis of randomized

controlled trials and prospective cohort studies. *CMAJ*. 2017;189(28):929–939. doi:10.1503/cmaj.161390; Pan A, Malik VS, Hao T, Willett WC, Mozaffarian D, Hu FB. Changes in water and beverage intake and long-term weight changes: results from three prospective cohort studies. *Int J Obes (Lond)*. 2013 Oct;37(10):1378–1385. doi:10.1038/ijo.2012.225.

13 Bolhuis DP, Lakemond CMM, de Wijk RA, Luning PA, de Graaf C. Consumption with large sip sizes increases food intake and leads to underestimation of the amount consumed. *PLoS One*. 2013;8(1):e53288. doi:10.1371/journal.pone.0053288.

14 Dennis EA, Dengo AL, Comber DL, et al. Water consumption increases weight loss during a hypocaloric diet intervention in middle-aged and older adults. *Obesity (Silver Spring)*. 2010;18(2):300–307. doi:10.1038/oby.2009.235.

15 Illescas-Zarate D, Espinosa-Montero J, Flores M, Barquera S. Plain water consumption is associated with lower intake of caloric beverages: cross-sectional study in Mexican adults with low socioeconomic status. *BMC Public Health*. 2015;15:405. doi:10.1186/s12889-015-1699-0.

16 Stroebele-Benschop N, Dieze A, Hilzendegen C. First come, first served. Does pouring sequence matter for consumption? *Appetite*. 2016;105:731–736. doi:10.1016/j.appet.2016.07.011.

17 Camps G, Mars M, de Graaf C, Smeets PA. Empty calories and phantom fullness: a randomized trial studying the relative effects of energy density and viscosity on gastric emptying determined by MRI and satiety. *Am J Clin Nutr*. 2016;104(1):73–80. doi:10.3945/ajcn.115.129064.

Day #21: Embrace the 80/20 Rule

1 Birch LL, Fisher JO, Davison KK. Learning to overeat: maternal use of restrictive feeding practices promotes girls' eating in the absence of hunger. *Am J Clin Nutr*. 2003;78(2):215–220.

2 Jansen E, Mulkens S, Emond Y, Jansen A. From the Garden of Eden to the land of plenty: restriction of fruit and sweets intake leads to increased fruit and sweets consumption in children. *Appetite*. 2008;51(3):570–575. doi:10.1016/j.appet.2008.04.012.

3 Coelho do Vale R, Pieters R, Zeelenberg M. The benefits of behaving badly on occasion: Successful regulation by planned hedonic deviations. *J Consum Psychol*. 2016;26(1):17–28. doi: 10.1016/j.jcps.2015.05.001.

4 Mead NL, Patrick VM. The taming of desire: unspecific postponement reduces desire for and consumption of postponed temptations. *J Pers Soc Psychol*. 2016;110(1):20–35. doi:10.1037/a0039946.

Day #22: Master Special Occasions

1   Diaz-Zavala RG, Castro-Cantu MF, Valencia ME, Alvarez-Hernandez G, Haby MM, Esparza-Romero J. Effect of the holiday season on weight gain: a narrative review. *J Obes.* 2017; ID 2085136. doi:10.1155/2017/2085136.
2   US Department of Health and Human Services and US Department of Agriculture. *2015–2020 Dietary Guidelines for Americans.* 8th ed. Washington, DC; 2015;34.
3   De Witt Huberts JC, Evers C, Ridder D. Double trouble: restrained eaters do not eat less and feel worse. *Psychol Health.* 2012;28(6):686–700. doi:10.1080/08870446.2012.751106.

Day #23: Stay on Track

1   Kuijr RG, Boyce JA. Chocolate cake. Guilt or celebration? Associations with healthy eating attitudes, perceived behavioural control, intentions and weight-loss. *Appetite.* 2014;74:48–54. doi:10.1016/j.appet.2013.11.013.
2   Mantzios M, Wilson JC. Making concrete construals mindful: a novel approach for developing mindfulness and self-compassion to assist weight loss. *Psychol Health.* 2014;29(4):422–441. doi:10.1080/08870446.2013.863883.
3   Kiernan M, Moore SD, Schoffman DE, et al. Social support for healthy behaviors: scale psychometrics and prediction of weight loss among women in a behavioral program. *Obesity (Silver Spring).* 2012;20(4):756–764. doi:10.1038/oby.2011.293.
4   Ross K, Qiu P, You L, Wing R. Characterizing the pattern of weight loss and regain in adults enrolled in a 12-week internet-based weight management program. *Obesity (Silver Spring).* 2018;26(2):318–323. doi:10.1002/oby.22083.
5   Thomas JG, Bond DS, Phelan S, Hill JO, Wing RR. Weight-loss maintenance for 10 years in the National Weight Control Registry. *Am J Prev Med.* 2014;46(1):17–23. doi:10.1016/j.amepre.2013.08.019.
6   LaRose JG, Leahey TM, Hill JO, Wing RR. Differences in motivations and weight loss behaviors in young adults and older adults in the national weight control registry. *Obesity (Silver Spring).* 2013;21:449–453. doi:10.1002/oby.20053.

Day #24: Step It Up

1   Curioni CC, Lourenco PM. Long-term weight loss after diet and exercise: a systematic review. *Int J Obes (Lond).* 2005;29:1168–1174. doi:10.1038/sj.ijo.0803015.
2   2018 Physical Activity Guidelines Advisory Committee. *2018 Physical Activity Guidelines Advisory Committee Scientific Report.* Washington, DC: US Department of Health and Human Services, 2018.

3   Zhang J, Brackbill D, Yang S, Becker J, Herbert N, Centola D. Support or competition? How online social networks increase physical activity: a randomized controlled trial. *Prev Med Rep.* 2016;4:453–458. doi:10.1016/j.pmedr.2016.08.008.

4   Bigliassi M, Karageorghis CI, Hoy GK, et al. The way you make me feel: psychological and cerebral responses to music during real-life physical activity. *Psychol Sport Exerc.* 2018. doi:10.1016/j.psychsport.2018.01.010.

5   How much physical activity do adults need? Centers for Disease Control and Prevention website. https://www.cdc.gov/physicalactivity/basics/adults/index.htm. Updated August 13, 2018. Accessed August 14, 2018.

6   Stiles VH, Metcalf BS, Knapp KM, et al. A small amount of precisely measured high-intensity habitual physical activity predicts bone health in pre- and post-menopausal women in UK Biobank. *Int J Epidemiol.* 2017;6:1847–1856. doi:10.1093/ije/dyx080.

7   Rosique-Esteban N, Díaz-López A, Martínez-González MA. Leisure-time physical activity, sedentary behaviors, sleep, and cardiometabolic risk factors at baseline in the PREDIMED-PLUS intervention trial: a cross-sectional analysis. *PLoS One.* 2017;12(3):e0172253. doi:10.1371/journal.pone.0172253.

8   Stamatakis E, Kelly P, Strain T, et al. Self-rated walking pace and all-cause, cardiovascular disease and cancer mortality: individual participant pooled analysis of 50 225 walkers from 11 population British cohorts. *Br J Sports Med.* 2018;52:761–768.

9   Bhammar DM, Angadi SS, Gaesser GA. Effects of fractionized and continuous exercise on 24-h ambulatory blood pressure. *Med Sci Sports Exerc.* 2012;44(12):2270–2276. doi:10.1249/MSS.0b013e3182663117.

10 Feig EH, Lowe MR. Variability in weight change early in behavioral weight loss treatment: theoretical and clinical implications. *Obesity (Silver Spring).* 2017;25(9):1509–1515. doi:10.1002/oby.21925.

11 Yoga—benefits beyond the mat. *Harvard Health Publishing.* https://www.health.harvard.edu/staying-healthy/yoga-benefits-beyond-the-mat. Published February 2015. Accessed March 5, 2018.

12 Kaewkannate K, Kim S. A comparison of wearable fitness devices. *BMC Public Health.* 2016;16:433. doi:10.1186/s12889-016-3059-0.

13 Tigbe W, Granat M, Sattar N. Time spent in sedentary posture is associated with waist circumference and cardiovascular risk. *Int J Obes.* 2005;41(5). doi:10.1038/ijo.2017.30.

Day #25: Sleep Deep

1   Wu Y, Zhai L, Zhang D. Sleep duration and obesity among adults: a meta-analysis of prospective studies. *Sleep Med.* 2014;15(12):1456–1462. doi:10.1016/j.sleep.2014.07.018.

2   How much sleep do we really need? National Sleep Foundation website. https://sleepfoundation.org/excessivesleepiness/content/how-much-sleep-do-we-really-need-0. n.d. Updated 2018. Accessed March 3, 2018.

3   Al Khatib HK, Hall WL, Creedon A. Sleep extension is a feasible lifestyle intervention in free-living adults who are habitually short sleepers: a potential strategy for decreasing intake of free sugars? A randomized controlled pilot study. *Am J Clin Nutr.* 2018;107(1):43–53. doi:10.1093/ajcn/nqx030.

4   Spaeth AM, Dinges DF, Goel N. Effects of experimental sleep restriction on weight gain, caloric intake, and meal timing in healthy adults. *Sleep.* 2018;36(7):981–990. doi:10.5665/sleep.2792.

5   Miller MA, Kruisbrink M, Wallace J, Ji C, Cappuccio FP. Sleep duration and incidence of obesity in infants, children, and adolescents: a systematic review and meta-analysis of prospective studies. *Sleep J.* 2018;41(4):1–19. doi:10.1093/sleep/zsy018.

6   Sleep may trim neural connections to restore learning ability [press release]. National Institute of Mental Health; https://www.nimh.nih.gov/news/science-news/2017/sleep-may-trim-neural-connections-to-restore-learning-ability.shtml. Published February 20, 2017. Accessed March 3, 2018.

7   Sleep and sleep disorders. Centers for Disease Control and Prevention website. https://www.cdc.gov/sleep/index.html. Updated February 22, 2018. Accessed March 3, 2018.

8   St-Onge MP, Mikic A, Pietrolungo CE. Effects of diet on sleep quality. *Adv Nutr.* 2016;7(5):938–949. doi:10.3945/an.116.012336; Food and drink that promote a good night's sleep. National Sleep Foundation website. https://sleepfoundation.org/sleep-topics/food-and-drink-promote-good-nights-sleep. Updated 2018. Accessed April 22, 2018.

9   Steen J. We ask sleep experts whether warm milk can really help you fall asleep. *Huffington Post* website. https://www.huffingtonpost.com.au/2016/08/04/we-ask-sleep-experts-whether-warm-milk-can-really-help-you-fall_a_21444739/. Published Sept 8, 2016. Accessed February 20, 2018.

10 Lin HH, Tsai PS, Fang SC, Liu JF. Effect of kiwifruit consumption on sleep quality in adults with sleep problems. *Asia Pac J Clin Nutr.* 2011; 20(2):169–174.

11 St-Onge MP, Mikic A, Pietrolungo CE. Effects of diet on sleep quality. *Adv Nutr.* 2016;7(5):938–949. doi:10.3945/an.116.012336.

12 St-Onge MP, Mikic A, Pietrolungo CE. Effects of diet on sleep quality. *Adv Nutr.* 2016;7(5):938–949. doi:10.3945/an.116.012336.

13 Howatson G, Bell PG, Tallent J, Middleton B, McHugh MP, Ellis J. Effect of tart cherry juice (Prunus cerasus) on melatonin levels and enhanced sleep quality. *Eur J Nutr*. 2012;51(8):909–916. doi:10.1007/s00394-011-0263-7.

14 Losso JN, Finley JW, Karki N, et al. Pilot study of the tart cherry juice for the treatment of insomnia and investigation of mechanisms. *Am J Ther*. 2018;25(2):e194–e201. doi:10.1097/MJT.0000000000000584.

15 St-Onge MP, Mikic A, Pietrolungo CE. Effects of diet on sleep quality. *Adv Nutr*. 2016;7(5):938–949. doi:10.3945/an.116.012336.

16 Light-emitting e-readers before bedtime can adversely impact sleep. Brigham Health website. https://www.brighamandwomens.org/about-bwh/newsroom/press-releases-detail?id=1962. Published December 22, 2014. Accessed March 10, 2018.

Day #26: Unplug to Unwind

1 Cruikshank T. *Meditate Your Weight*. New York: Harmony; 2016:43.

2 Geiker NRW, Astrup A, Hjorth MF, Sjodin A, Pijls L, Markus RC. Does stress influence sleep patterns, food intake, weight gain, abdominal obesity and weight loss interventions and vice versa? *Obes Rev*. 2017;19(1):81–97. doi:10.1111/obr.12603.

3 Kiecolt-Glaser JK, Habash DL, Fagundes CP. Daily stressors, past depression, and metabolic responses to high-fat meals: a novel path to obesity. *Biol Psychiatry*. 2015;77(7):653–660. doi:10.1016/j.biopsych.2014.05.018.

4 Kushlev K, Dunn EW. Checking email less frequently reduces stress. *Comput Human Behav*. 2015;43:220–228. doi:10.1016/j.chb.2014.11.005.

5 Zeidan F, Martucci KT, Kraft RA, McHaffie JG, Coghill RC. Neural correlates of mindfulness meditation-related anxiety relief. *Soc Cogn Affect Neurosci*. 2014;9(1):751–759. doi.org/10.1093/scan/nst041; Goyal M, Singh S, Sibinga EMS, et al. Meditation programs for psychological stress and well-being: a systematic review and meta-analysis. *JAMA*. 2014;174(3):357–368. doi:10.1001/jamainternmed.2013.13018.

6 Cho H, Ryu S, Noh J, Lee J. The effectiveness of daily mindful breathing practices on test anxiety of students. *Plos One*. 2016;11(10):e0164822. doi:10.1371/journal.pone.0164822.

7 Cruikshank T. *Meditate Your Weight*. New York: Harmony; 2016:43.

8 Labbé E, Schmidt N, Babin J, Pharr M. Coping with stress: the effectiveness of different types of music. *Appl Psychophysiol Biofeedback*. 2007;32:163–168. doi:10.1007/s10484-007-9043-9.

9 Torres R, Ribeiro F, Duarte JA, Cabri JMH. Evidence of the physiotherapeutic interventions used currently after exercise-induced muscle damage: systematic review and meta-analysis. *Phys Ther Sport*. 2012;13(2):101–114. doi:10.1016/j.ptsp.2011.07.005.

10 Kim HJ. Effect of aromatherapy massage on abdominal fat and body image in post-menopausal women. *J Korean Acad Nurs.* 2007;37(4):603–612. doi:10.4040/jkan.2007.37.4.603.

Day #27: Love and Connect

1   Holt-Lunstad J, Smith TB, Layton JB. Social relationships and mortality risk: a meta-analytic review. *PLoS Med.* 2010;7(7):e1000316. doi:10.1371/journal.pmed.1000316.

2   Powell K, Wilcox J, Clonan A, et al. The role of social networks in the development of overweight and obesity among adults: a scoping review. *BMC Public Health.* 2015;15:996. doi:10.1186/s12889-015-2314-0.

3   Christakis NA, Fowler JH. The spread of obesity in a large social network over 32 years. *N Engl J Med.* 2007;357:370–379. doi:10.1056/NEJMsa066082.

4   Henning CH, Zarnekow N, Hedtrich J, Stark S, Türk K, Laudes M. Identification of direct and indirect social network effects in the pathophysiology of insulin resistance in obese human subjects. *PLoS One.* 2014;9(4):e93860. doi:10.1371/journal.pone.0093860; Komaroff A. Social networks can affect weight, happiness. *Harvard Health Publishing.* https://www.health.harvard.edu/blog/social-networks-can-affect-weight-happiness-201112163983. Published December 16, 2011. Accessed April 22, 2018.

5   Kushner RF, Blatner DJ, Jewell DE. The PPET study: people and pets exercising together. *Obesity (Silver Spring).* 2006;14(10):1762–1770.

6   O'Haire M. Companion animals and human health: benefits, challenges, and the road ahead. *J Vet Behav.* 2010;5(5):226–234. https://doi.org/10.1016/j.jveb.2010.02.002; Lippman F. *How to Be Well: The 6 Keys to a Happy and Healthy Life.* Boston: Houghton Mifflin Harcourt; 2018.

7   Xu W, Oei TP, Liu X, et al. The moderating and mediating roles of self-acceptance and tolerance to others in the relationship between mindfulness and subjective well-being. *J Health Psychol.* 2016;21(7):1446–1456. doi:10.1177/1359105314555170.

8   Pillay S. Greater self-acceptance improves emotional well-being. *Harvard Health Publishing.* https://www.health.harvard.edu/blog/greater-self-acceptance-improves-emotional-well-201605169546. Published May 16, 2016. Accessed April 22, 2018.

9   University of Maryland Medical Center. Laughter helps blood vessels function better. *ScienceDaily.* www.sciencedaily.com/releases/2005/03/050310100458.htm. Published March 16, 2005. Accessed January 29, 2018.

10 Strean WB. Laughter prescription. *Can Fam Physician.* 2009 Oct;55(10): 965–967.

11 Agroskin D, Klackl J, Jonas E. The self-linking brain: a VBM study on the structural substrate of self-esteem. *PloS One.* 2014;9(1):e86430. doi:10.1371/journal.pone.0086430.

12 Holt-Lunstad J, Smith TB, Baker M, Harris T, Stephenson D. Loneliness and social isolation as risk factors for mortality. *Perspect Psychol Sci.* 2015; 10(2):227–237. doi:10.1177/1745691614568352.

13 Holt-Lunstad J, Smith TB, Layton JB. Social relationships and mortality risk: a meta-analytic review. *PLoS Med.* 2010;7(7):e1000316. doi:10.1371 /journal.pmed.1000316.

14 Sirois FM, Kitner R, Kirsch JK. Self-compassion, affect, and health-promoting behaviors. *Health Psychol.* 2015;34(6):661–669. doi:10.1037/hea0000158.

15 Adams CE, Leary MR. Promoting self-compassionate attitudes toward eating among restrictive and guilty eaters. *J Soc Clin Psychol.* 2007;26(10): 1120–1144.

16 Forgiveness: your health depends on it. Johns Hopkins Medicine website. https://www.hopkinsmedicine.org/health/healthy_aging/healthy_connections /forgiveness-your-health-depends-on-it. Updated 2018. Accessed March 5, 2018.

Day #28: Stretch Your Horizons

1 Cell Press. Pure novelty spurs the brain. *ScienceDaily.* www.sciencedaily.com /releases/2006/08/060826180547.htm. Published August 27, 2006. Accessed March 7, 2018.

2 Pearson DG, Craig T. The great outdoors? Exploring the mental health benefits of natural environments. *Front Psychol.* 2014;5:1178. doi:10.3389 /fpsyg.2014.01178.

3 Razani N, Morshed S, Kohn MA, et al. Effect of park prescriptions with and without group visits to parks on stress reduction in low-income parents: SHINE randomized trial. *PLoS One.* 2018. doi:10.1371/journal.pone.0192921.

Day #29: Pursue Your Passion

1 Vallerand RJ. The role of passion in sustainable psychological well-being. *Psychol Well Being.* 2012;2(1). doi:10.1186/2211-1522-2-1.

2 Csikszentmihalyi M. *Flow: The Psychology of Optimal Experience.* New York: Harper Perennial Modern Classics; 2008.

3 Kobau R, Sniezek J, Zach M, et al. Well-being assessment: an evaluation of well-being scales for public health and population estimates of well-being among US adults. *Appl Psychol.* 2010. doi:10.1111/j.1758-0854.2010.01035.x.

4 Khullar D. Finding purpose for a good life, but also a healthy one. *New York Times.* January 1, 2018. https://www.nytimes.com/2018/01/01/upshot/finding -purpose-for-a-good-life-but-also-a-healthy-one.html. Accessed March 14, 2018.

Day #30: Start Each Day Anew

1   Killingsworth MA, Gilbert DT. A wandering mind is an unhappy mind. *Science.* 2010;330(6006):932. doi:10.1126/science.1192439.

2   Diener E, Chan MY. Happy people live longer: subjective well-being contributes to health and longevity. *Appl Psychol.* 2011. doi:10.1111/j.1758-0854.2010.01045.x.

3   Killingsworth MA, Gilbert DT. A wandering mind is an unhappy mind. *Science.* 2010;330(6006):932. doi:10.1126/science.1192439.

Index

About the Author

Lisa R. Young, PhD, RDN, CDN, is an internationally recognized nutritionist and portion control expert. She is an adjunct professor of nutrition at New York University, author, international lecturer, and media consultant. As a registered dietitian nutritionist in private practice, Young counsels adults and children on a wide variety of nutrition and health issues.

Dr. Young is the author of *The Portion Teller Plan: Eating, Cheating, and Losing Weight Permanently*, which was named one of the six best health books by the *Wall Street Journal* and *O, The Oprah Magazine*. She has authored peer-reviewed research articles as well as popular features on portion sizes and served as an adviser to the New York City Department of Health and Mental Hygiene on its various portion-control initiatives.

Major media outlets, including the *Wall Street Journal*, the *New York Times*, *USA Today*, the *Washington Post*, *Newsweek*, CNN, FOX, NBC, ABC, and CBS, routinely call on Dr. Young as an expert voice on nutrition, diet, wellness, and portion control. She appeared in the award-winning documentary *Super Size Me* and the BBC documentary series *The Men Who Made Us Fat*. The Israel Cancer Research Fund (ICRF) named Dr. Young a "Woman of Action."

Dr. Young received her doctorate and master's degrees in nutrition from New York University and her bachelor's degree in economics and health care administration from the Wharton School of the University of Pennsylvania. She lives in New York City.

www.drlisayoung.com

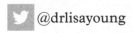 @drlisayoung   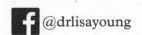 @drlisayoung   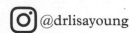 @drlisayoung